Dr Penny Stanway is an experienced doctor, medical author, journalist and broadcaster. She has written for newspapers including the Mail on Sunday and The Times, consumer magazines such as Parents and Woman's Weekly, and many professional journals. In addition, she has appeared on various television and radio programmes including GMTV, TV-AM and Woman's Hour, and has been Woman's Weekly's health columnist for thirteen years. Her other books include Breast is Best, Healing Foods for Common Ailments, The New Guide to Pregnancy and Babycare and The Natural Guide to Women's Health.

FIRST BABY
AFTER 30 ...
OR 40?

DR PENNY STANWAY

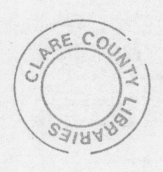

ORION

An Orion Paperback
First published in Great Britain in 1999 by
Orion Books Ltd,
Orion House, 5 Upper St Martin's Lane,
London WC2H 9EA

Fourth impression
Reissued 2004
Revised edition

A CIP catalogue record for this book
is available from the British Library.

ISBN: 0 75281 595 4

Printed and bound in Great Britain by
Clays Ltd, St Ives plc

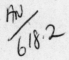

AN/
618·2

CONTENTS

PREFACE TO THE SECOND EDITION

The big changes in women's behaviour already under way when I wrote the first edition of *First Baby After* 30 . . . *or* 40? four years ago have continued apace. The age at which women are having their first baby continues to creep up. Waiting till 30 or older is now so common that even though the total number of babies born in the UK is shrinking year on year, the number born to women over 30 is steadily growing.

SO WHAT'S GOING ON?

More and more women in their 20s and 30s are enjoying freedom, independence and wealth without the responsibility of a family. They often use this time to progress in their career; some have their own home; and many have spare money to spend on entertainment, clothes, eating out and holidays.

Men too are relishing life as singletons or DINKY (Double Income No Kids Yet) couples. They are pleased to defer parenthood and are increasingly likely to balk at the idea of having a baby and, perhaps, becoming the sole breadwinner until they are established in their careers, with enough money to continue their lifestyle while paying a mortgage currently supported by two incomes. Many know that while a woman may *say* she'll go back to work soon after giving birth, she may in her heart of hearts want to stay with the baby. And this is indeed what tends to happen, with women often returning to work years later than they originally envisaged – and then maybe only part-time.

However, deferring parenthood encourages fertility problems. And while we've always known that female fertility decreases with age, recent research proves that men too become less fertile over the years, so that by 45, for example, they are five times less likely to father a baby.

All this helps explain why fewer babies have been born each

year since 1991. In England and Wales, for example, the birth rate in 2001 was the lowest since records were first collected in 1924, with fewer than 600,000 births. The average woman now has only 1.6 babies, compared with 2.9 in 1964 – a huge social change in just 35 years. Knowing they'll probably ever have only one or two children, many women opt to wait ten or so years before starting a family. These changes are mirrored throughout the world – in Italy and Russia, for example, the average woman has only 1.2 babies, in France, 1.7, in Ireland, 1.9 and in Bangladesh, 3.3.

Major changes are clearly afoot, so let's look at births over 30 more closely.

INTRODUCTION

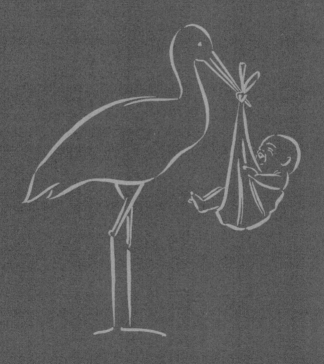

Women who have their first child after 30 or 40 have special concerns and questions and expect particular rewards and joys. This book will guide you step by step through the whole process – from making your decision, to the birth ... and beyond.

YOU'RE IN GOOD COMPANY

Today's woman is more likely than her sisters at any time in recorded history to have her first baby after 30. Changing lifestyles, opportunities and expectations are altering childbearing patterns too. Most women have children but the proportion of those who don't is growing in most western countries. The average woman not only has her first baby later than her counterpart of even just ten years ago but also ends up with a smaller family. In several western countries the birth-rate is now lower than the death-rate.

WHAT NATURE INTENDED FOR WOMEN

A woman can conceive and give birth right up to around her menopause – but only if she is fertile.

Most girls become fertile soon after starting periods, at an average age (in developed countries) of nearly 13. And women become infertile when they stop releasing eggs – usually shortly before the menopause. This occurs at an average age of 51, though in some women it's later, which means they could become pregnant in their 50s.

The stark facts are that a young woman's fertility begins to decline in her late 20s and that this decline gathers momentum from her mid-30s on. As a result, a sizeable proportion of the increasing

Today's woman is more likely than her sisters at any time in recorded history to have her first baby after 30

number of women who postpone their first baby finds conception – and successful pregnancy – difficult, if not impossible.

AND MEN?

The average man makes millions of sperms each day and although their number and quality may decline after 50, he can probably father a child well into old age. While he needs energy and desire to find, attract and have sex with a partner, he doesn't need the health and strength to carry a baby through pregnancy, give birth and breastfeed!

Well-known men to hit the headlines as older fathers are actors Clint Eastwood, a father again at 66, and Anthony Quinn, at 81.

THE MENOPAUSE – NOT THE END?

Natural conception after the age of 50 is highly unusual. However, some women become very unexpectedly pregnant years after their menopause. The UK record is held by a woman of 60. Modern reproductive technology is developing so fast that the menopause need no longer necessarily mean the end of fertility. Assisted conception now enables some women in their 50s and 60s to have babies, so the possible age range for pregnancy is widening, albeit by artificial means, some of which are unacceptable to some people.

For example, in 1997, the same year as a 12-year-old in the UK gave birth to a daughter, a Southern Californian woman of 63 became the world's oldest mother. And in 1998, a 55-year-old woman had quadruplets in the US, and a woman of 60 became the UK's oldest woman to be a first-time mother.

CHANGES IN FIRST BABIES' MOTHERS' AGES

According to the Office for National Statistics for England and Wales, both the proportion and the number of births over 30 are increasing.

Figures for 2001 reveal that for the very first time, more first babies (49,894) were born to married women aged 30–34, than to any other age band. (There are no figures for unmarried women, even though more babies are now born to single mums than married ones!) The next most popular age band was 25–29, with 49,076 babies. Third came 20–24-year-olds with 22,305. And 19,489 babies were born to over-35s.

All this represents a great leap forward in the number of first births to over-30s compared with even just four years before, in 1997. Then, 25–29 was by far the most popular age band, with 63,044 first babies born, and while there were 48,015 first births to women aged 30–34, only 15,782 babies were born to over-35s.

There's been an even bigger shift since 1987, when first babies were born to only 33,284 women aged 30–34, and only 8,907 over-35s.

In summary, the number of women having first babies over 30 was half as high again in 2001 as just 14 years before, in 1987. And the number having first babies over 35 more than doubled.

These are big changes in 14 years, with the trend very clearly favouring older motherhood.

These changes in the UK are closely mirrored by changes in the US, where a quarter of first-time births are now to women over 30. The changes are similar in Australia. And wherever they are, they well and truly capture public attention, as judged by the huge interest in those female show-biz personalities who have their first child in their 40s.

So first-time motherhood in the 30s and 40s is clearly becoming more popular (or, at least, more common). And with women in their 50s and 60s giving birth, albeit only a very few and usually with medical help, the fact that more women are giving birth for the first time later in life raises few eyebrows.

WHY ARE WOMEN DELAYING MOTHER-HOOD?

More women are waiting until their 30s or 40s because they are:
• Becoming more highly educated and desirous of further

experience while they are independent.
- Establishing a career.
- Using safe, acceptable, reliable contraception.
- Seeking a desirable partner, perhaps because an earlier relationship has ended in divorce.
- Waiting to commit themselves to a man before he becomes the father of their child.
- Waiting for their man to commit himself to a long-term relationship, and to fatherhood.
- Enjoying the status quo and not wanting to rock the boat (or cradle!).
- Deciding earlier to be child-free and then changing their mind.
- Choosing to copy what so many men have always done, by starting a family in their 30s or 40s rather than in their 20s or even teens.

Actively delaying motherhood is one thing, but the longer you wait, the less fertile you and your man become, and the longer it's likely to take for you to get pregnant.

YOUR UNIQUE EXPERIENCE

Whatever your age or reason for having – or thinking of having – your first baby in your 30s or 40s, this book sets out to trigger debate, answer questions and help you make the most of your experience, opportunity and potential.

Use it to help you assess the pros and cons. Bring yourself up to date on preparing for pregnancy and what to do if you prove less fertile than you hoped. And learn how best to look after yourself and your developing child, and how to manage or avoid common problems.

I'll also discuss special tests and suggest how to prepare for and manage your baby's birth. Finally, there's a section on feeding your baby and caring for yourself as a mother, as well as a mention of alternative ways of mothering.

And I wish you *bon voyage* in your journey.

CHAPTER ONE

Deciding on a baby

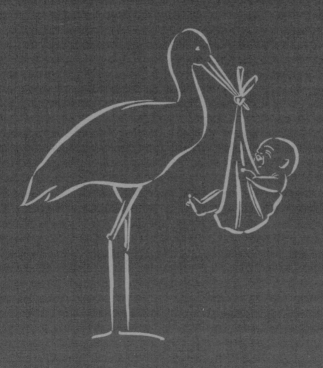

Couples in earlier generations had much less choice and often became parents nine months after the honeymoon. In many ways this made things much easier.

Nowadays, for better or for worse, nature and desire no longer dictate what happens, and most of us have to make a positive decision if we want a baby. This may not be as straightforward as it sounds.

THE DECISION-MAKING PROCESS

Some people are born to decision-making: they thrive on considering options and picking the best. Others find it time-consuming, hard work or even exhausting. And a few decide first one thing, then another, frequently changing their minds and making themselves and others frustrated and upset.

If you are finding it difficult to decide about a baby, or hard to stick with your decision, this five-point scheme may help:
1. Think through your options.
2. Explore the motivations lying behind each one.
3. Weigh up the pros and cons of each.
4. Let go – or 'mourn' – the ones you discard.
5. Affirm and celebrate your decision.

Points 1 and 2 are touched on in this chapter and the rest are covered in the next.

YOUR OPTIONS – A BABY ... MAYBE ... OR NOT?

As women and men go through their 30s or 40s, the issue of having children usually becomes increasingly important.

What you decide depends partly on whether you and your partner have a committed relationship.

You may find yourself in one of these situations:

- **You and your partner both want a baby** – but don't know when.
- **You want a baby but can't get pregnant or keep miscarrying** (see Chapter Four). Older women in particular can't necessarily expect to have a baby just because they want one.
- **Your partner doesn't want a baby**. If so, you can either go along with him, or try to change his mind. If you can't live with the idea of remaining child-free, you may even choose to look for a new partner who feels the same way as you. Some women use subterfuge by allowing contraception to fail; in others the unconscious takes over and makes them 'forget' the Pill. Some women whose partners use a condom secretly 'borrow' another man and suggest their partner's condom must have had a hole. Tricking a man into becoming a father – or even bringing up another man's child – is hardly the best way of embarking on family life; it's unfair and some would say it's unforgivable, but it has always happened. Turning the tables, a man who wants a baby but whose partner doesn't has little, if any, choice – unless he were to damage his condom and rely on his pregnant partner refusing an abortion.

> A *few women opt to be a lone parent by borrowing a fertile, willing man*

- **You want a baby but don't have a partner**. Your best bet is to carry on trying to find a man who wants a family. A few women opt to be a lone parent by borrowing a fertile, willing man or arranging for insemination with donated semen. A partnerless man who wants a baby has no comparable option!
- **You don't want a baby**. You may or may not change your mind. However, a tiny but relatively fast-growing percentage of women is choosing to remain childless – or 'child-free'. If current trends continue, one in five women in the UK now in their 20s will never have children. And a recent Mintel survey (on 'Pre-Family Lifestyles') found that 17 per cent of 20–34-year-olds didn't ever want a baby. So a sizeable minority of young women have no plans for children. Some even reinforce their

choice by being sterilised! In 1996 around 400 young, childless women opted for this operation on the NHS and many more went privately. NHS gynaecologists are reluctant to sterilise women under 30 in case they want the operation reversed later. Sterilisation reversal is technically possible in only four women in five.

> **One in five women in the UK now in their 20s will never have children**

As for when to start a pregnancy, this will depend partly on how urgently you want a baby. It may also depend on your age, the likely number of fertile years you have remaining (see pages 12 and 41) and your career plans.

KNOWING YOUR OWN MINDS

It isn't always easy to know what *you* want to do about having a baby, let alone what your partner wants!

However, empathic listening can be a useful tool in making up your minds. Make time to listen to your inner voice and your feelings about starting a family. Recognising and acknowledging such feelings may help you decide.

Listen to your partner too. To do this effectively, put your feelings and beliefs aside. Identify his emotions – from what he says, how he says it, his body language and behaviour. Then, most important, let him know you care by suggesting what you think he's feeling, and allowing him time to respond with what he actually *is* feeling.

WHY NOW?

Most couples want a family. Before reliable contraception existed there was little choice over when to start. We now have much more control but even so, surveys suggest that one in two pregnancies is unplanned – though not necessarily unwanted.

Most of us, whatever our age, have mixed reasons for wanting a baby – or not. Some are buried in our unconscious mind and it's these – rather than contraceptive failure or lack of planning – that underlie many unplanned pregnancies. For it can be tempting, at some unconscious level, to use contraception ineffectively – to, as it were, play Russian roulette with your chance of conceiving – so you might get pregnant without ever consciously planning to do so.

If you're trying to make up your mind, clarify things by asking, 'Why now?' Here are some possible reasons:

You feel broody.
You both want a family and see no reason to wait.
You want to be a mother.
You want to celebrate or cement your relationship – or save an ailing one. (The latter reason is a very bad one for creating a new life.)
Your partner wants a baby.
You are worried about your biological clock.
You're in a new relationship and want to 'give' a baby to your man.
You think it's time for a career break.
You are comfortable enough financially.
Your work and lifestyle make a baby seem feasible for the first time.

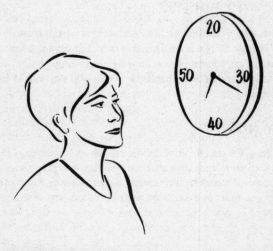

You've made your mark at work and have some job security.
You want to stop work.
You desperately long for a child.
You want to be pregnant and the centre of attention.
You need to succeed at something.
You are following your family pattern.

FOLLOWING FAMILY PATTERNS

Some families have a tradition of each generation being a particular age when they have their first baby. For example, if your female relatives – mother, grandmother and sister – had their first babies after 30 and seemed happy, you may want to follow their example. The same goes for your man and his relations. But things aren't always so simple. For example, if your mother had her first child after 30 or 40 but seemed *un*happy, you might decide to be a younger mother instead. And if your mother was disappointed, frustrated or angry not to have had a career or freedom because she had a baby in her teens or 20s, you might opt for later motherhood.

AGE AND WHAT IT MEANS

Everyone has different ideas about age and what it means. These ideas can be so powerful that they influence how you feel about yourself and your life.

If you are trying to decide about having a baby, it may help to look at what the various ages when you could become a parent mean to you. For example, however old you are, do you believe people in their 30s are no longer young? Do you think middle age begins at 40? Or do you believe that how old you feel and whether you enjoy life are all in the mind?

It is worth noting that children seem to benefit from parents who are not bowed by any imagined weight of the years in themselves but let a youthful nature leaven the wisdom of maturity.

HOW MUCH LONGER IS LEFT BEFORE YOUR MENOPAUSE?

Deciding when to have a baby might be easier if you knew how many fertile years stretched ahead. However, this is easier said than done because some women are less fertile than others. And some women's fertility declines and comes to a halt relatively rapidly. A premature menopause (defined as one before 40) happens to one woman in 100.

The G-Test is a sensitive new blood test which may prove very useful in this respect. Developed in the UK, this is the first to reveal how well a woman's ovaries are working and whether she can afford to wait to get pregnant or should start trying without delay.

It involves having an ultrasound scan to check the ovaries and a blood test for follicle-stimulating and luteinising hormone levels, followed by a nasal spray of a pituitary-stimulating drug (buserelin), and then daily hormone tests on days two, three and four of the menstrual cycle. The results of these tests indicate whether the ovaries have a good, sub-optimal or poor response to hormonal stimulation. These responses equate with the level of fertility.

A woman with a good response is likely to have a minimum of two fertile years ahead, although one of the experts who devised the test advises that even if a woman over 35 has a good response, she shouldn't delay if she wants a baby.

A woman of any age with a poor response and who wants a child is advised to start trying without delay.

The G-Test is now available in some fertility clinics, and may be particularly useful if you want to delay motherhood, but know that the women in your family tend to have a premature menopause. An over-the-counter saliva-test kit based on similar principles may eventually become available too.

WORK AND CAREER IMPLICATIONS

If you work, then whatever your age it makes sense to think of the implications of having a baby.

Although most women choose to stay home with very young

children, many work part-time as their children grow up. Some opt for full-time work – possibly even straight after their official maternity leave.

If you work, your baby will need excellent care. But however good this may be and however well your child does, you'll sacrifice some of the rewards of full-time motherhood.

Many large organisations have now made themselves more flexible and 'parent-friendly' – mainly to attract and retain high-quality staff – by allowing such arrangements as job-shares, reduced hours, part-time work, flexitime, or even a few years out to raise young children.

Discuss your options with your employer and any professional organisation or union to which you belong. And remember to consider the implications that stopping work may have on financial responsibilities such as your pension and mortgage.

YOUR FUTURE FAMILY

Making plans for the future with a child also means taking others into account. Not only will you continue to be someone's 'child' yourself and, possibly, a sibling too, but you'll also be a parent and, with your partner, a co-parent. Having a child will proba-

> *Having a child will bind you and your partner in a way that even separation or divorce will never dissolve*

bly forge deeper relationships between your two families. All this means that your hopes and dreams, successes and failures, and long-term relationships and duties will affect many more people's lives than before. And having a child will bind you to your partner in a way that even later separation or divorce can never dissolve.

HOW BIG A FAMILY DO YOU WANT?

A healthy, fertile 30-year-old can probably have any size family she wants. At 40 her declining fertility may mean she has to limit her ideas. If you would like only one or two children it may not much matter when you start. But if you want more and have a choice, it's wise to start sooner rather than later.

WHAT ARE YOUR IDEAS ABOUT FAMILIES – AND DOES YOUR PARTNER AGREE?

Don't forget that you and your partner may have different views. While one, for instance, may expect a large family, the other may dream of giving an only child heaps of attention. Your expectations (both conscious and unconscious) of family life may also differ and it's wise to discuss things early on.

COULD YOU COPE WITH PREGNANCY AND PARENTING AS A SINGLE PARENT?

The answer is you can't know ahead of time. Of course almost every woman would prefer to bring up her child with the loving support of a partner committed to her and her child. But this isn't always possible. You could lose your partner through separation, divorce or death. Or you may become pregnant by someone who isn't committed to you.

Although they may say it's tough, many lone parents have the strength and skill to give their baby and themselves much of what they both need and, if necessary, to arrange work and child-care so they can earn enough to support themselves. Many also have a network of supportive friends. For those who don't have all this, the UK's welfare state provides basic support.

UNPLANNED PREGNANCIES

An unplanned pregnancy is a relatively frequent occurrence among women in their 30s and 40s. Their reactions depend partly on their circumstances. Some are delighted; some are shocked but eventually come to terms with the idea and go on to welcome the child and feel positive about motherhood. Others are dismayed and consider abortion, perhaps because their lives are so settled or their income so tight that they or their partners find it hard to accept any disruption.

Women in their 40s are less fertile than when they were younger but most can still get pregnant. There's always been talk (unproven as far as I know) of a very temporary boost to fertility just before the menopause, with 'the ovaries having a final fling'. And even when a woman reaches menopausal age, pregnancy is a possibility for a year after her last period – if this was after 50 – or for two years if before 50.

Considering your options and motivations is the first step in deciding if and when to have a baby. The next, perhaps, is looking at the pros and cons.

CHAPTER TWO
The pros and cons

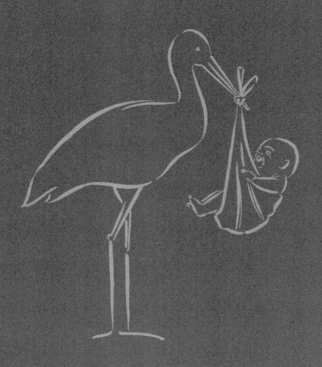

Exploring the advantages and disadvantages of a first baby after 30 or 40 is interesting and valuable. It can also be very emotional.

Three people will be most affected – you, your partner and the child you may bring into the world – though your decision will inevitably touch the lives of others too.

Some of the consequences may be beneficial, others detrimental – and some will simply make life different.

POSSIBLE ADVANTAGES FOR YOU, YOUR PARTNER AND YOUR RELATIONSHIP

Privilege, joy and pride. Having a child can be a privilege and a joy. Many parents feel proud and some say that having a child and being a good parent are among the most important things they ever do.

Enjoyment of your growing child. A child may be delightful, amusing, interesting, thought-provoking, thoughtful, helpful, compassionate, instructive and fascinating. Most parents benefit hugely, with more personal enjoyment than they could ever have foretold.

A particularly deep love-bond. Raising your own child offers a new dimension unequalled by caring for other children. However much you love someone else's child, almost everyone experiences a deeper, more lasting love for their own flesh and blood.

Challenge, wisdom and maturity. Children's behaviour through the various ages and stages of development provides parents with many opportunities to increase their repertoire of understanding, tolerance, compassion and creativity. And responding to this challenge by broadening your outlook and improving your management skills could give you the opportunity and potential reward of becoming a wiser, more mature human being.

More self-confidence and management skills. Your life experience will hopefully enable you to manage your life more effectively than when you were younger. This could ease the practicalities and emotional stresses of parenting. And you're more likely than a younger woman to benefit from the experience of friends who've already embarked on parenthood.

A young outlook. Being with a child, sharing activities and providing an interested, listening ear for questions, hopes and fears keeps parents aware of young interests and viewpoints. This gives you the opportunity to relearn the importance of play and to widen your social circle by mixing with the parents of your child's friends; also, contact with younger parents can be stimulating and refreshing.

> *Many parents who have their first baby relatively late say they feel younger at heart than their peers*

Many parents who have their first baby relatively late say they feel younger at heart than their peers.

Less breast, ovary and womb cancer. Having a baby at any age makes a woman less likely to develop breast, ovary or womb cancer. The later you have your first child, the greater the reduction in ovary-cancer risk.

A longer life. A fascinating 1997 study revealed that female centenarians were more likely than women who died in their 70s to have given birth in their 40s. Unfortunately, this doesn't mean that having a child in your 40s will make you live to 100!

A later menopause. Mothers have a later menopause on average than do childless women, so their high pre-menopausal oestrogen level protects their bones from the increased post-menopausal mineral loss for longer. This means that having a child can delay the onset of osteoporosis (fragile bones due to bone mineral loss). In fact, each child delays the average woman's menopause by about five months. Moreover, women who give birth after 40 have a later menopause than women who do so before 40.

A deepening relationship with your partner. Your experience as parents will challenge your relationship. Meeting this challenge constructively – perhaps with the benefit of goodwill, effective relationship skills and support from others – will give your love a chance of becoming stronger. Also, your partner may be better at sharing you with a baby if he's already had several years of a one-to-one relationship.

Better sex in pregnancy. One survey found that women over 35 felt more positive about sex during pregnancy than did those in their 20s.

A chance to train, earn and progress at work. Having a baby in your 30s or 40s gives you the chance to advance your career before starting a family. It also allows you to collect a nest-egg or start buying a house first.

A chance to help your partner financially. Delaying a family until your 30s or 40s might allow you to support your partner financially while he studies for professional or other qualifications or starts a business. You might consider this to be a sound invest-ment for your future family.

Hope for the future. A baby is a symbol of life continuing from one generation to the next. A baby also gives his or her parents a lasting stake in this future – a way of carrying something of them-selves and their families down the centuries.

POSSIBLE ADVANTAGES FOR YOUR CHILD

More chance of being breastfed. The children of women who give birth over 35 are far more likely to be breastfed (see page 122) than those of mothers in their 20s. They are also likely to be breastfed for longer.

A wiser, more mature mother. Hopefully your child will benefit from the experience, wisdom and maturity you bring from over three or four decades of life. Some people even think older mums are better mums, although this is hotly disputed and much obvi-ously depends on the individual. However, what you can claim for sure is that as an older parent you'll have had time to learn the vital truth that love and attention are more important to a child than material possessions.

A more sensitive mother. Your child stands to gain if your life experience has made you relatively self-aware – or at least more

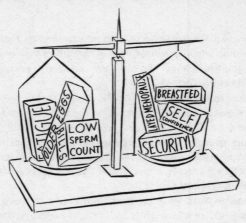

interested in being so. This is because awareness of your own feelings, needs, attitudes, motivations and behaviour should make you more sensitive to all these things in your child.

Better educational and behavioural development. One survey found that children of older mothers scored higher in certain educational and behavioural tests. For example, 4-year-olds understand more words if they have older mothers. Psychologists say this is partly because older mothers talk and listen to their young children more than younger ones do.

Temperamental differences. A recent study found that children of older mothers tend to be more persistent and self-confident.

Financially secure parents. A child may know no different – and, of course, money can't buy happiness – but parents who are financially stable can make life more comfortable in material terms.

POSSIBLE DISADVANTAGES FOR YOU, YOUR PARTNER AND YOUR RELATIONSHIP

Delayed conception. You could take slightly longer to conceive than a younger woman.

Higher risk of fertility problems or actual infertility. The older you are, the higher your risk of being unable to conceive at all.

More pregnancy problems. There is a slightly higher risk of certain pregnancy problems, including miscarriage, high blood pressure, diabetes, ectopic pregnancy (see page 107) and pre-term labour. Your risk of having a stillborn baby is also raised, though it remains small.

Longer labour. The older you are when you have your first baby, the longer your labour is likely to be.

Higher risk of Caesarean operation. If you have your first baby in your 30s or 40s you're more likely to have a Caesarean operation. One study, for example, showed that over-35s having their first babies had twice as many Caesareans as did younger women!

More fatigue. Parents of young children complain more about feeling tired than anything else. Broken nights are arguably harder in a woman's 40s than in her 20s. And a huge amount of physical work, time and emotional energy goes into bringing up a child, especially if you work too. Even when children first leave home – perhaps to go to university or college – many parents still spend a lot of time servicing them, albeit from afar. All this is true for any parent – but some women who have their first baby in their 30s or 40s seem more tired than younger women. And you'll be a lot older when your late teen or adult child needs your ongoing support.

Less independence, spontaneity and free time, and more responsibility. Having a child almost inevitably means that for a very long time you'll have less independence and less time for yourself. Once you have a baby, popping out for a swim, meeting a friend for a drink, or looking round the shops calls for pre-planning. Some women find it's harder to give up this freedom when they've been used to it throughout their 20s or 30s.

Children need looking after and their needs are often so urgent that they must be met before you meet your own. Indeed, young children may sometimes seem to control the whole household and, as they grow older, want a say in such things as what the family eats and what everyone watches on TV.

Less time alone with your partner. You'll have less time to be alone with your partner – unless, that is, you're in the unusual situation of having a nanny. A way round this is to arrange regular baby-sitting – for example, by joining a baby-sitting circle.

Disruption to your relationship. Most couples find that having their first baby is the single most disruptive event in their lives together. Although this isn't something most people consider beforehand, it makes every sense to acknowledge the possibility and plan how to manage it. Some men become so used to a one-to-one relationship that they find it difficult to adjust when a baby arrives.

More bills. You'll have many more bills to pay, especially if your child is privately educated, continues into further education, needs help to start a business, or needs a home in his or her 20s and makes little, if any, contribution. If you have a baby in your 30s, this financial burden will continue at least into your late 40s and perhaps well into your 50s. If you have a baby in your 40s, the bills will continue past retirement.

Estimates of the cost of raising a child vary. A recent one for a child from birth to 17 in the UK was £50,000. Another which took into account the cost of expensive toys, child-care, private education and two foreign holidays a year, was £5,000 for the first five years of a first child's life, and £250,000 (1997 prices) up to the end of university. Child-care alone can cost over £6,000 a year, which is one reason why nearly one in two working women relies on informal child-care from family and friends.

More breast and ovary cancer. The older a woman is when she has her first child, the higher is her risk of developing breast or ovary cancer later. Delaying motherhood until you are in your 30s increases your risk of pre-menopausal cancer by 63 per cent and of postmenopausal cancer by 35 per cent compared with having a baby when you are younger. And the later you have a baby, the greater is your risk of ovary cancer.

Loss of contact with work colleagues. If you become a full-time mother, you'll miss your work and colleagues, but you can keep in touch with them socially and develop a new network of friends.

Less career progression. Many women either don't want to or can't put work first when they become mothers. This can mean that if they eventually return to work, they may find themselves on a slower track or be more likely to be blocked by a 'glass ceiling'.

Less chance of being a young granny. When your child has children, you may not have as much energy to spare for playing active games, going on outings and baby-sitting.

POSSIBLE DISADVANTAGES FOR YOUR CHILD

Higher risk of chromosomal abnormalities, including Down's syndrome. The later into her 30s and 40s a woman becomes pregnant, the higher is her baby's chance of Down's syndrome. This condition causes a characteristic physical appearance and learning difficulties, and results from there being an extra chromosome in each body cell. Other, rarer genetic abnormalities become more likely too.

This may be because:

- Her eggs have deteriorated with age.
- Her partner's sperm – if he is the same age or older – for some reason makes a genetically abnormal baby more likely. (A French study of sperm donors showed that babies with genetic fathers over 39 were three times as likely to have Down's syndrome as those with fathers under 35.)
- Either egg, sperm or both have been damaged by an environmental hazard such as radiation from X-rays.

It's important to put the increased risk into perspective. Overall, the Down's syndrome risk is:

1 in 2,000 if you are 20	1 in 100 at 40
1 in 1,400 at 25	1 in 50 at 45
1 in 1,000 at 30	1 in 20 at 46
1 in 350 at 35	

Although at 40 the risk is 1 in 100, this means that 99 babies are normal, so the odds are still extremely good. And it's interesting that the risk of the first baby of an older woman having Down's syndrome is less than that of a second or third child born to a woman the same age.

You can have screening tests for Down's syndrome in pregnancy (see Chapter Eleven).

Higher risk of kidney and breast cancer. Children of older mothers have a slightly increased risk of developing a kidney cancer called Wilm's tumour. Fortunately, this can often be successfully treated, particularly if the symptoms (such as a swelling or pain in the abdomen) are spotted early. Girls with older mothers are also very slightly more likely to develop breast cancer in later life. As for any woman, it's sensible for them as adults to be breast-aware – familiar enough with their breasts to spot changes that might indicate cancer.

> *The risk of the first baby of an older woman having Down's syndrome is less than that of a second or third child born to a woman the same age*

Lowered fertility. Sons born to women in their late 30s and 40s are more likely, as adults, to have fertility problems from poor quality sperm. This risk rises with the age of their mother at their birth, and may be caused by genetic changes in ageing eggs.

Embarrassment. Most children are occasionally embarrassed by their parents. It goes with the turf. The children of relatively older parents who behave or dress in an old-fashioned way may have what they consider to be perfectly good reason to be embarrassed!

A tired or unwell mother. As a child grows, having a mother who's always tired isn't much fun. Some people naturally age faster than others or consider feeling tired and unwell an inevitable part of ageing. However, as far as I know there's no biological reason for a healthy mother in her 30s and 40s to feel any different from one in her 20s, though bringing up a child can in itself be physically and emotionally tiring.

An unfit mother. As the years pass most people become less fit, mainly because they don't look after themselves by exercising regularly and eating a healthy diet. The downside for a child is having a mother who's too easily tired to play active games, go for walks, and so on.

A mother who doesn't understand young people. Some people lose touch with what's going on around them as they get older. A child whose parent is out of touch with their generation's behaviour, beliefs and attitudes may feel that he or she doesn't understand them or, worse, isn't interested.

HOW OTHERS MAY BE AFFECTED

The birth of a new baby affects many lives. There'll be new grandparents, great-aunts and uncles, aunts, uncles, cousins and, perhaps, godparents, perhaps a step-family and more besides. So your decision affects not only you and your partner but others too in what is a unique and important way. You are making your clan bigger – and most clans love that.

ADAPTING TO CHANGE

Things will obviously change a great deal when your baby comes along and the way you adapt will make all the difference. You'll need to:
- Recognise the difference between how things were and what now is.
- Allow yourself time and space to experience and explore how you feel about losing the old and gaining the new.
- Work out ways of adapting to and making the most of what's new and, most important, practise those ways which seem most useful.
- Celebrate your new situation.

Some people consider the pros and cons of a baby and then decide it's not for them.

But if you, like most, choose to go ahead, now's the time to celebrate one of the most important decisions you'll ever make. Your health and happiness are major determinants of your wellbeing and that of your baby.

So when the time is right – perhaps even now – you can start preparing for pregnancy.

CHAPTER THREE
Getting ready to start a baby

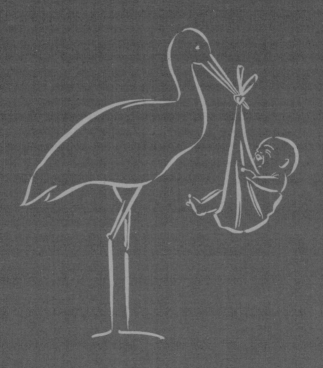

You and your partner are the raw material from which your baby will develop. There's a lot about ourselves we can't alter, but a preconception health and fitness programme allows you to increase your chance that the sperm and egg that hit it off at conception are strong and well formed.

It also makes a woman more likely to have a healthy pregnancy and a man better able to support his partner.

And the best time to start is well before you stop using contraception.

YOUR FOOD

Get in the habit of eating a healthy, balanced diet to supply the protein, carbohydrate, fat, vitamins, minerals, plant hormones, pigments and all the other phyto-nutrients and essential fatty acids you need. Go for:

- Five or more daily helpings of a variety of salads, vegetables (raw or only lightly cooked) and fruits. Include peas, beans, lentils, nuts and seeds. A 'helping' is a small bowlful or a piece of fruit. Wash, scrub or peel salads, vegetables and fruit to remove pesticide traces, or eat organic. Farmers have government guidelines for agricultural pesticide use, but a Soil Association spokesman has said, '... it's impossible to protect consumers from organophosphate residues simply by requiring growers to use pesticides more carefully'.
- At least two helpings a week of fish, including one of oily fish (salmon, sardines, trout, mackerel, pilchards, herring, for example). However, both now and during pregnancy, avoid eating shark, swordfish and marlin, and limit your weekly consumption of tuna to no more than one steak (140g cooked or 170g raw), or two medium-size cans (140g drained weight per can). This is because the levels of mercury are relatively high in these fish, and a high mercury intake could affect your baby's nervous

system. If you don't like oily fish, consider a supplement of fish oil (not fish *liver* oil, whose high vitamin A level is potentially unsafe in pregnancy).

- Mostly wholegrain foods (such as wholemeal bread, wholegrain breakfast cereals, brown rice) rather than refined-grain foods (white bread and rice, many breakfast cereals).
- Less fatty food. Many of us eat too much animal and other largely saturated fats (dairy food, hard cooking and spreading fats, most red meat).
- Foods rich in folic acid (green leafy vegetables, citrus fruit, beans, peas, potatoes, oranges, fortified bread and cereal, nuts, yeast extract – such as Marmite, and dairy food).

FOLIC ACID SUPPLEMENTS

You need a folic acid supplement even if you eat a healthy diet. Begin when you start seriously considering a baby – preferably at least a month before you start trying – and continue until the first 12 weeks of pregnancy are over (or longer, see page 70). A lack of folic acid very early in pregnancy – perhaps before you even know you are expecting – can lead to a baby having a neural tube defect (spina bifida – a spinal defect which can paralyse, or anencephaly – a skull and brain defect which kills).

A woman planning her first baby needs a 400mcg (microgram) tablet of folic acid each day. A woman who has previously miscarried a baby with a neural tube defect (or lost such a baby) needs a 4mg (milligram) tablet each day, 5mg tablets will do if 4mg ones are unavailable.

OTHER SUPPLEMENTS

Most doctors currently consider that there's no need for the average healthy woman to take any other supplements during the pre-conception months.

However, if either you or your partner continues to have an unhealthy diet, to be underweight because of eating too little, to smoke, or to drink a lot of alcohol – or if you find it difficult to conceive or have had several miscarriages – it may be sensible to take a vitamin and mineral supplement.

If it's your problem, take a daily multi-vitamin and mineral supplement formulated especially for pre-conception and pregnancy (details from your pharmacist or doctor, or see page 136).

If it's your partner's problem, he should take a multi-purpose multi-vitamin and mineral supplement.

WEIGHT: SLIMMING AND PUTTING ON THE POUNDS

If you weigh too much or too little, do something about it as far ahead of starting a baby as possible, because achieving and maintaining a healthy weight takes time and effort. Maintaining a healthy weight for your height and build is important because:

- Being overweight can reduce fertility in both sexes. An Australian study of women who were 20 per cent overweight and unable to conceive for an average of five years reported that losing some or all of their excess weight enabled three out of five to conceive!
- One in three newly pregnant British women is overweight and one in six obese. However, an overweight woman is more likely to miscarry, possibly before she even knows she is pregnant.
- Very over- or underweight men probably eat an unhealthy diet with insufficient nutrients to form healthy sperms and feel optimally fit and well.
- Being severely underweight may prevent egg-release and so prevent conception.
- A woman who is underweight even before she conceives has a greater chance of having a low birth-weight baby.
- A good nutrient supply helps prevent babies being malformed and miscarried, and keeps a woman feeling well.
- Researchers now believe that poor maternal nutrition at particular stages of fetal development increases a baby's risk of certain diseases as an adult. These include high blood pressure, type-1 diabetes, and cardiovascular disease (which causes heart attacks and strokes).

ALCOHOL

Men and women are more fertile if they avoid too much alcohol. Not only can alcohol harm sperms and eggs but it can also damage a newly formed baby – and a woman trying for a baby may be pregnant for some weeks without knowing. US researchers who recently observed 5,000 pregnant women noted that even five units of alcohol a week in the first ten weeks quadrupled the risk of miscarriage.

The problem, however, is that experts don't know for sure how much is too much. Also, women and their babies vary in their response to alcohol, and any danger is increased by smoking and caffeine consumption.

So what should *you* do about alcohol when trying for a baby?

You may decide to cut it out completely. This is safest but some find it attractive only if they or their partner has fertility problems or they've had one or more miscarriages. You could limit alcohol to, for example, a maximum of one or two drinks for you, and two or three for your partner, just once or twice a week.

COFFEE

There's no evidence that moderate amounts of coffee (see page 72) reduce fertility. And while a few studies suggest that larger amounts reduce fertility, the majority don't.

EXERCISE

Almost everyone feels better if they get their bodies moving and their hearts and lungs working faster for at least half an hour a day. There's an extra shine and vitality in their eyes and clarity and glow in their skin. Their weight tends to stabilise at a healthy level. They feel happier and more optimistic. And they are more likely to keep well.

Exercise boosts the circulation, which is good for the ovaries, testes, womb, penis and every other part of the body – and good news both for conception and carrying a baby successfully.

The habit of regular exercise also makes most people feel more like sex, which is a help when trying to get pregnant.

DAYLIGHT

Spend time in the open air each day to get daylight on your skin and – without looking directly at the sun – your eyes. Even in northern latitudes the amount of ultra-violet and other rays absorbed just through your face will help keep you happy and healthy. Top up your light requirement in the summer. In winter, if you can spare only a little time, go outside at midday.

Having sufficient sunlight has special relevance for older women because it:

- Boosts fertility by stimulating the body's hormone-controller – the hypothalamus – in the brain.
- Produces vitamin D and oestrogen which boost reserves of calcium and other minerals in the bones, enabling them to stay stronger and resist fractures in later life.
- Helps prevent winter depression (seasonal affective disorder, or SAD).

SMOKING

If I give only one piece of profes-sional advice to women thinking of a baby, it's, 'Be a non-smoker!'. So if you're already a smoker, be sure to stop, or cut right down, at least three months before even trying for a baby.

A woman who smokes ten or more a day takes nearly twice as long to conceive as does a non-smoker

Handling and smoking cigarettes, and inhaling nicotine may be temporarily relaxing, comforting or otherwise pleasurable, and you may think smoking is 'cool' but it's also detrimental to both men's and women's health and fertility.

A woman who smokes ten or more a day takes nearly twice as

long to conceive as does a non-smoker. Smoking increases the risk of early miscarriage – perhaps before you even know you are pregnant. And if you continue to smoke into pregnancy and beyond it has special dangers. For more information and tips on stopping, see pages 82–83.

STRESS

A certain amount of stress is stimulating and good. Sometimes, though, stress becomes too much to handle effectively and makes us unwell. Many women in their 30s and 40s lead such busy, responsible lives that they are particularly liable to suffer from stress. See pages 82–86 for practical help with stress relief and management.

PREPARING YOUR RELATIONSHIP

Considering the importance, the hugeness of the task and the time it takes to bring up a child, it's extraordinary that we have no formal preparation for parenthood. We could, of course, call our very lives a preparation. But is it possible to build our relationship so as to prepare for being a threesome?

I think it is. Two of the best ways are learning and practising empathic listening skills and encouraging each other more. Another is to learn management skills so you can work as a team.

WHEN TO STOP USING CONTRACEPTION

The Pill. Ex-Pill users take longer to conceive than women giving up other forms of contraception, and over-30s may take up to a year. So, ideally, stop the Pill at least three months (and some experts recommend up to 12 months) before you want to conceive. In the meantime use a condom, diaphragm or the sympto-thermal method (perhaps with the help of a saliva microscope or electronic ovulation monitor, see page 44).

This Pill-free time allows your body to correct Pill-induced changes in its levels of vitamin B (including folic acid), iron and zinc; restore regular periods and ovulation; and, if you were on the progestogen-only Pill, it makes an ectopic pregnancy (see page 107) less likely.

Don't worry, though, if you happen to conceive while on the Pill. Studies confirm that this doesn't harm a baby, though it makes sense to stop as soon as possible. Older women who conceive while on the Pill have a slightly increased chance of twins.

The coil. Have a hormone-releasing coil removed several months before you want to conceive so as to lower your risk of an ectopic pregnancy. Have a copper coil removed six months before, to allow your body to shed stored copper. High copper levels have been linked with premature labour, low birth-weight and neural tube defects.

Your body may need a month or two to restore regular periods and ovulation after a non-copper, non-hormone coil comes out.

Hormone implants. Have a hormone implant removed several months before you want to conceive.

THE BEST TIME TO HAVE SEX FOR GETTING PREGNANT

A man is fertile all the time, but the average woman only around the time of ovulation (see page 42).

It's interesting that men may fancy women more around ovulation. They respond to the scent of a woman's hormones at this time of the month with a massive 50 per cent increase in testosterone! It is also well known that women are most interested in sex around ovulation time.

CHOOSING YOUR BABY'S SEX

Many parents want to be able to choose a boy or girl but doctors aren't yet confident enough about the safety to the baby of test-tube gender-selection techniques, and most are understandably unwilling to use gender-selective abortion for social reasons (though they may consider it if a baby's risk of a sex-linked genetic disease such as muscular dystrophy is high).

HOME METHODS

An 80 per cent success rate is claimed for the diet below. The other methods are unproven but harmless and possibly worth trying.

For a girl:

- Loose underpants and trousers for your partner.
- Frequent sex from the end of your period up to the day before ovulation. Vaginal mucus is relatively acid at this time and favours the relatively acid-resistant 'female' sperms.
- Days 7–9 are the most likely in the average cycle for conceiving a girl. Avoid the day of ovulation and the one after (days 14–15 in the average cycle), when the vagina is relatively alkaline.
- Douche half an hour before sex with a teaspoon (5ml) of white wine vinegar in a pint (600ml) of warm water to make the vagina more acidic.
- You should avoid orgasm as this releases alkaline mucus.
- You should eat a diet rich in calcium and magnesium (eg dairy food, eggs and nuts) and low in sodium and potassium (eg salt, meat and fish) for at least six weeks (more information from Jonathan Hewitt, Liverpool Women's Hospital, Crown Street, Liverpool L8 7SS).
- Aim to conceive in the spring, from March to the end of May.
- Find a toy boy! Older women married to younger men have more girls than boys.

For a boy:

- Your partner should wear tight-fitting underpants.
- He can try having a cold shower or immersing his testicles in a cold bath each day, as well as avoiding hot baths.
- It might help if he either avoids very high-stress situations or uses effective stress-management strategies. This is based on the fact that pilots, racing drivers and certain other men in high-stress occupations have more girls than boys.
- If you're coping with a recent stressful event, postponing trying for a baby may boost your chances of having a boy.
- He should cut down on alcohol and smoking.

- Avoid penetrative sex from the day your period ends until the day you ovulate. In the first half of your cycle the vaginal mucus is relatively acid and more likely to destroy the weaker 'male' sperms.
- Have sex on the day of ovulation – day 14 in the average cycle – and the day after, when your vaginal mucus is relatively alkaline and friendly to male sperms.
- Douche with a dessertspoon (10ml) of sodium bicarbonate in a pint (600ml) of warm water half an hour before sex to make the vagina more alkaline.
- You should try for orgasm as this releases alkaline mucus.
- You should eat a diet rich in sodium and potassium but low in calcium and magnesium for at least six weeks before conceiving (see above for more information).
- Aim to conceive in the autumn, from September to the end of November.
- Marry an older man! Women younger than their partner by six years or more seem to have more boys.

MEDICAL TECHNIQUES

You may or may not think these methods are acceptable:

Sperm labelling and sorting – a technique currently being researched in the US which dyes sperms' DNA (genetic material) and gives them an electrical charge. Bigger 'female' gynaesperms have an X chromosome with more DNA, smaller 'male' androsperms a Y, with slightly less DNA. Gynaesperms take up more dye and charge, and separate out when passed between electrically charged plates. Sperms of the desired gender are used either for test-tube fertilisation followed by implantation of one or more embryos into the womb, or for artificial insemination. This technique offers an 85 per cent chance of having a girl, or a 65 per cent chance of having a boy.

Test-tube fertilisation, cell sampling of embryos to select one or more of the desired gender, and implantation into the womb.

Amniocentesis or chorionic-villus sampling to discover the sex of the baby in the womb, then abortion of a baby of the unwanted gender.

AROMATHERAPY OILS

It's lovely to be massaged with an oil containing fragrant essential plant oils. However, some are not advised for women who might be pregnant and so are best avoided as soon as you stop using contraception (see page 81).

MEDICINES

If you need medication, let your doctor know before a prescription is written that you are trying to get pregnant and discuss over-the-counter medication with the pharmacist. Some drugs are best avoided now but safe treatments can nearly always be substituted.

Avoid vitamin and mineral supplements other than those formulated for pregnancy.

Check that any herbal remedies you use are suitable for women who might unknowingly be pregnant.

DRUGS

It's best to avoid the dangerously and coyly named 'recreational' drugs such as cannabis, ecstasy and cocaine at any time, but especially now.

ENVIRONMENTAL HAZARDS

X-rays. If you need an X-ray, tell the doctor, radiographer or dentist you are thinking of becoming pregnant – in case you already are! You should schedule a non-emergency X-ray for the first week of your cycle and have extra radiation protection.

Pesticides. Exposure to biocides – weedkillers (herbicides) and pesticides (insecticides and fungicides) – may endanger eggs and sperms, and damage, or even kill, unborn babies. Any potentially poisonous household, garden or agricultural biocide should carry prominent warnings and instructions. Unless you are sure it's safe, don't inhale its vapour, and keep it off your skin. This applies to flea sprays and fly-catching papers too. If you live within a quarter of a mile (400 metres) of crops being sprayed, then unless you know that the product is a harmless fertiliser, or a biocide which isn't dangerous to humans, go away for the day. Afterwards, avoid walking near newly sprayed fields and inhaling any morning or evening mist hanging over them.

Burning plastics. Avoid breathing smoke from burning plastics; if these contain PVC (polyvinylchloride) their smoke may contain dangerous PCBs (polychlorinated biphenyls).

Stripping paint. If you want to strip or otherwise disturb paint which might contain lead (which includes many household paints used before the 1960s), and you are, or might be, pregnant, stay away until the job is done and the paint dust or debris has been thoroughly cleared. Inhaled or swallowed lead from the dust or fumes of disturbed lead-containing paint collects in a pregnant woman's bones and is readily transferred into her unborn baby's body where it can lead to brain damage and other health problems. Information on testing for lead and stripping lead paint safely is available from the Paintmakers Association (see page 135).

Vapour from solvents, glues, etc. Avoid inhaling vapour from solvents, paints, thinners, glues, marking pens and perchlorethylene (a dry-cleaning fluid).

Chemicals at work. If you work with chemicals, check that your employer observes any necessary safety precautions for women who might be – or already are – pregnant. Some potentially hazardous chemicals are mentioned above. Others include mercury, cytotoxic drugs, formaldehyde, glutaraldehyde and anaesthetic gases. The highest risks are found in the chemical, plastics, pharmaceutical, rubber and textile industries, as well as in market gardening and farming.

RUBELLA IMMUNISATION

Rubella (German measles) in pregnancy can seriously damage an unborn baby, so if you have never been immunised ask your doctor for a simple blood test to see if you are immune. If you are not, you can be immunised now. However, it's crucial to avoid pregnancy for a month afterwards.

INFECTIONS THAT MAY DAMAGE YOUR BABY (SEE PAGE 108)

All babies are precious but an older woman may be particularly eager to save a newly conceived baby from a potentially dangerous yet possibly avoidable infection.

So, if you can, steer clear of children and adults who are unwell and either have or have reason to think they are about to get chickenpox, rubella, flu or other common viral infections which could endanger an unborn baby. And avoid crowded places when possible. Obviously, though, this advice is the counsel of perfection and may not be achievable in real life.

TOXOPLASMOSIS

Infection with protozoa called *Toxoplasma gondii* in pregnancy can make you miscarry or may damage your baby. So as you could be pregnant for some days or weeks without realising, take precautions against this infection now:

* Wear rubber gloves when handling soil.
* Wash salads, vegetables and fruit before eating.
* Don't eat raw or undercooked meat.
* Wash your hands after handling raw meat.
* Ask someone else to empty your cat's litter tray – or wear rubber gloves.
* Disinfect your cat's litter tray each day.
* Avoid contact with sick cats.

LISTERIOSIS

This very rare infection can lead to miscarriage, stillbirth or preterm birth. Since you might become pregnant at any time, avoid it from now on by not eating:

* Pâté made from meat, fish or vegetables.
* Soft, mould-ripened cheeses (such as Brie and Camembert) and blue-veined cheeses. Experts in the US also warn against

feta cheese. Non-blue hard cheeses, and soft cheeses such as cottage, cream, spread, ricotta, Mozzarella and mascarpone, are safe.
- Soft-whip ice cream.
- Unpasteurised milk.
- Pre-cooked poultry.
- Cooked chilled food – unless reheated thoroughly.
- Prepared salads – unless washed thoroughly.
- Underdone meat.

A SPECIAL WORD FOR SHEPHERDESSES

Avoid contact with ewes and lambs in the lambing season to prevent infection with *Chlamydia psittaci*, which can trigger miscarriage. And don't handle the clothing of anyone who has been in contact with lambs or ewes.

Last but not least, get medical advice if you develop an unusual vaginal discharge or pelvic pain. Certain infections (some sexually transmitted infections such as chlamydia and gonorrhoea) may reduce fertility. An overgrowth of bacteria normally present in the vagina (bacterial vaginosis) may, once you get pregnant, encourage late miscarriage or premature birth (see pages 93 and 103).

Continue your pre-conception health programme until you're pregnant and then on into pregnancy. If you aren't pregnant after a few months of trying, you can give nature a helping hand by using the tips in the next chapter.

CHAPTER FOUR

Fertility matters

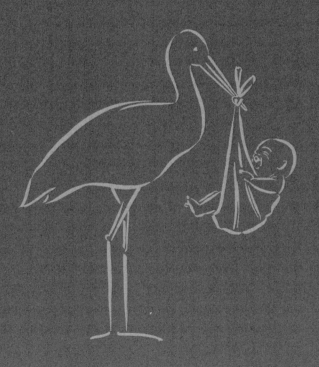

T he average woman is at peak fertility in her early 20s, her biological clock then makes her increasingly less fertile from the late 20s to the menopause.

THE EGG SUPPLY

The average woman's egg supply – fixed when she is an unborn baby – dwindles hundreds at a time in each menstrual cycle, and also during pregnancy, breastfeeding and when on the Pill. The number falls from around a million at birth to 250,000 at puberty and around 1,000 at the menopause. One thousand eggs is too few to enable her to have periods any more. Indeed, even when she is around 45, her eggs are already so few that her periods start to become irregular.

When a woman has only about 25,000 eggs remaining – which for the average woman is at 37 – she loses eggs twice as fast. And the fewer eggs she has – and the older they are – the less fertile she is. For example:

- A 35-year-old woman takes twice as long to conceive as one aged 25.
- A 38-year-old woman who has unprotected sex has only a quarter of the chance each month of conceiving and eventually having a healthy baby compared with a woman under 30.
- While five out of six couples of all ages have no problem starting a baby, the picture is different if the woman is in her 30s or 40s. In the US half of all women aged 35–45 have difficulty conceiving or carrying a baby to term. And it's thought that only three or four in every 100 women aged 44 can conceive and bear a healthy baby.
- Among certain religious groups that don't use contraception, the average age of a woman having her last child is 40–41.

All this has important implications for any woman wondering when to have her first baby. If she waits for some years she may have to try longer to conceive – or she may even be unable to become pregnant at all.

A SPECIAL SITUATION

If you have radiotherapy of an ovary or surgery to remove one ovary before you are 30, your menopause is likely to be seven years early, at an average age of 44, and your fertility will probably decline relatively fast before this too. This may make you decide not to wait too long to have a baby.

If you need surgery for an ovarian cyst it's worth asking the surgeon if it's possible to conserve the ovary and just remove the cyst, rather than remove the whole ovary.

AND MEN?

Add to the woman's situation the fact that men also become less fertile as their sperm count and quality decline with the passing years, and you can see that there's a very real problem for some couples who postpone parenthood. Indeed, the older you both get and the later you leave trying for your first baby, the more concerned and disappointed you'll be if your periods keep appearing. And you may feel sad, angry or frustrated at being unable to plan such a significant event, especially if you're used to being in control.

WHEN ARE YOU MOST FERTILE?

In normal circumstances a man is fertile all the time but a woman's cycles make her most fertile around ovulation. The woman with an average-length cycle ovulates on day 14 (counting the first day of her period as day 1). She is likely to be fertile on days 10–15 inclusive and particularly so on days 13–15.

However, the length of normal, regular, ovulatory cycles in different women varies from 24 to 32 days. Also, researchers have recently suggested that many women routinely ovulate several times in each menstrual cycle. As ovulation usually precedes the onset of menstruation by 14 days, a woman with a short, 24-day, cycle will probably ovulate on day 10, and a woman with a long, 32-day one, on day 18.

An egg must be fertilised within 24–36 hours. Ejaculated sperms generally survive for up to 72 hours (though some live for five days in 'fertile' mucus – see below). So the most fruitful time for sex is generally from 72 hours before to 36 hours after ovulation.

> *The most fruitful time for sex is generally from 72 hours before to 36 hours after ovulation*

Nature isn't always this predictable, though, and some women have been known to experience 'bunny-rabbit ovulation' – ovulating unexpectedly, like rabbits, in response to sex.

Clearly, if you want to have sex when you have the best chance of conceiving, it helps to know when you are most likely to ovulate.

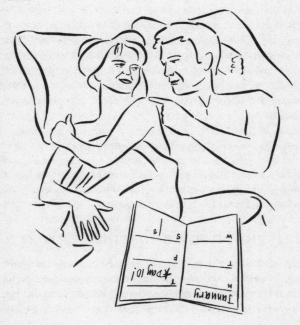

PREDICTING AND DETECTING OVULATION

Keep a period diary for several months. If your cycles are regular, you can then work out when you're likely to be most fertile each month.

Check your vaginal mucus. This becomes thinner, clearer and much more plentiful, slippery and stretchy in the few days before ovulation. Stretch it between your finger and thumb. If you are fertile it will form a long, elastic string. Ovulation generally occurs within 24 hours (sometimes 48) of peak mucus production; the amount of mucus decreases afterwards.

Use an ovulation predictor kit from a pharmacist a few days before you expect ovulation. A colour change in the paper stick dipped in your urine shows whether you're making enough luteinising hormone for conception to be possible.

Use an electronic ovulation predictor monitor (see page 136). This stores and collates information about your hormone levels over several cycles. When you insert a urine-moistened dipstick into the monitor it beams a red light when you are fertile, yellow when you might be, and green when you're not.

Watch out for a new ovulation prediction device – a modern version of an existing technique with which you examine your saliva through a simple microscope. Two or three days before ovulation the salivary oestrogen and progesterone levels are such that they combine with the salt naturally present to form a distinctive fern-like pattern of crystals. However, researchers say the original microscope test is unreliable, and it remains to be seen whether its modern equivalent will be any better – so you may not want the bother of doing it.

DIY METHODS FOR BOOSTING FERTILITY

Any couple finding it difficult to have a baby can take many practical, safe and largely unintrusive steps to optimise their natural fertility. It's important not to become stressed or obsessive about these methods however. You may find that they act as daily reminders of your continuing lack of fertility and as such may make you anxious or disappointed, or even dampen your sexual desire. If following any of these DIY tips makes one or both of you upset or starts spoiling your relationship, take a break – it may be just what you need!

Also remember that, in retrospect, these methods may turn out to be unnecessary or unhelpful, either because you'll conceive naturally in time, or because you won't be able to conceive without medical assistance or even, perhaps, at all.

FOR BOTH OF YOU:

Follow Chapter Three's advice. In particular, stop smoking (or, at the very least, cut down) and give up or limit alcohol. Both of these make early miscarriage more likely, and repeated early miscarriages – before you even know you're pregnant – are easily confused with an inability to conceive. Also, make sure you both eat a healthy diet with fresh salads, fruit and vegetables, including root vegetables, as well as nuts, seeds, beans, wholegrains and (for non-vegetarians) meat, fish and shellfish. This provides plenty of vitamins C and E, selenium and zinc, all especially important for nourishing sperms and eggs and helping sperms swim. Even a slight lack of zinc can reduce a man's testosterone level, sex drive and sperm count. Recent research suggests that even a small amount of alcohol (five units a week) can lower a woman's fertility.

Avoid any foods to which you are sensitive. The best way to identify a food sensitivity is to stop eating the suspect food for three weeks. If your symptoms disappear, reintroduce the food to see if they return. If so, do two more of these challenges to be quite sure. Get professional help if necessary to ensure that your diet remains nutritionally sound. If an elimination and repeated challenge trial makes you think you are sensitive to gluten (a protein in wheat, oats, barley and rye), blood tests and a small bowel biopsy (done via a swallowed tube) can confirm your suspicions. Gluten sensitivity is a recognised cause of infertility.

Have intercourse two or three times a week and every day of the week before ovulation – but only once a day!

Have intercourse when you wake in the morning, as most women ovulate in the afternoon and it may help for sperms to arrive first!

Relax (see page 80); being stressed-out can prevent ovulation and lower the sperm count.

Eat organic produce. A small proportion of some salads, vegetables and fruits consistently fails tests for safe levels of agricultural pesticide residues, and certain pesticides can lower the sperm count and lead to miscarriage.

FOR WOMEN:

Take a pregnancy mineral and vitamin supplement (see page 136).

Take a daily dose of evening primrose oil.

FOR MEN:

Take a multi-mineral and vitamin supplement. Researchers are studying whether a high-dose vitamin E supplement might boost male fertility. Whether a supplement of vitamins C and E and beta-carotene (a type of vitamin A) might help male infertility could depend on the problem: a recent survey found that if semen contained sperm auto-antibodies, it was likely to have relatively high levels of vitamin E but low levels of beta-carotene.

Avoid beer, as plant oestrogens and certain other ingredients may depress your sperm count.

Avoiding tight underpants and jeans is no longer advised. Recent research demonstrated no differences in semen in men wearing boxer shorts and those wearing briefs.

OCCUPATIONAL HAZARDS

Chemicals. Take the recommended safety precautions if you work with industrial or agricultural chemicals.

Ionising radiation. Female health workers and air crew exposed to ionising radiation should consult the doctor at work; it could be better to arrange now for the lower exposure limit usually assigned only when pregnancy is declared.

Heat exposure from driving and welding. Men who do long hours of driving might consider a break or change of job until their partner conceives; the prolonged, immobile seated position heats their testes, which can cause fertility problems. Men such as welders whose jobs involve actual heat exposure might find a long break or a job change helps too.

Stressful jobs. Having a long break or change from a high-stress job, or using effective stress-management strategies, can benefit both men and women.

Others. Women exposed to textile industry dust may benefit from a prolonged break or change of job, as may those who work as dental-surgery assistants.

WHEN TO SEEK PROFESSIONAL HELP

30–35 – seek help if you don't conceive after a year of regular, frequent sex.

Over 35 – seek help after six months.

POSSIBLE FERTILITY TESTS AND INVESTIGATIONS

Women: a physical examination and a blood test for your 'mid-luteal' progesterone level on day 21 of your cycle to check you are ovulating. Blood tests for other hormones may also be necessary. You may be offered a trans-vaginal ultrasound scan (see page 100); laparoscopy (examination of ovaries, tubes and womb via a viewing tube passed through the abdominal wall); and, possibly, X-rays of womb and tubes, a look inside the womb and a womb-lining biopsy. A blood test can provide chromosomes for analysis.

Men: a physical examination and two semen tests. A normal count is 30–120 million sperm per millilitre of semen, with 60 per cent normally formed and 60 per cent active after two hours. If there is an abnormal count the test is repeated 4–6 weeks later and sperm antibody and strength tests done. Blood tests can indicate hormone levels and provide chromosomes for analysis, and some men have a testis biopsy.

Both: a blood test for coeliac disease (sensitivity to gluten, a cereal protein) and, if positive, an intestinal biopsy. Gluten sensitivity is associated with fertility problems in men and women and there may be no other obvious signs.

FERTILITY TREATMENTS

Forty per cent of fertility problems stem from the woman, 30 per cent from the man, and 30 per cent are unexplained. Often more than one factor is involved. Very often women who think they are infertile are actually miscarrying time and time again without realising. A common and treatable cause for recurrent miscarriage is the production of antibodies which trigger clots in the placenta. The good news is that this can be treated (see page 96). Three out of four women who are not ovulating regularly have polycystic ovary syndrome, with irregular or absent periods, and perhaps acne and excess body hair. Many of them are overweight. Before accepting any treatment for fertility problems, be sure you know the likely success rate, as well as the risk of problems to you and your baby both now and later.

FOR WOMEN:

- Weight loss, a healthy low-carbohydrate diet, and daily exercise may help if you are overweight or obese, and tests reveal a lack of ovulation, plus polycystic ovaries. This is because your lifestyle may well be causing insulin resistance, a condition that can affect every part of the body, including the ovaries. You are overweight if your BMI (body mass index) is over 25, obese if it's over 30. Indeed, all women who are having assisted conception treatment and are overweight have a 75 per cent better chance of conceiving if they lose weight. Work out your body mass index as follows: take your weight (in kilograms); next multiply your height (in metres) by itself; then divide your weight by this 'height squared' number.
- Hormone therapy with clomiphene to stimulate egg release

(known as superovulation). However, researchers suspect this may trigger the growth of cancer in the breasts or ovaries, so it's important to have a breast check first, and to think twice if you have a family history of breast or ovary cancer. Also, clomiphene stimulation should be done only if ultrasound scans of the ovaries are done during treatment.

- Surgical removal of eggs and subsequent fertilisation with the partner's sperm in a test tube and transfer of the embryo to the woman's cervix or womb (IVF-ET – *in vitro* fertilisation plus embryo transfer).
- Micro-surgery can sometimes clear blocked Fallopian tubes.
- Removal of a fibroid or surgical destruction of patches of endometriosis (medical treatment for endometriosis does not improve the chance of pregnancy).
- ZIFT (zygote intra-Fallopian transfer) involves surgically removing eggs, mixing them with the partner's sperm, and putting them in a Fallopian tube.
- GIFT (gamete intra-Fallopian transfer) involves surgically removing eggs, mixing them with the partner's sperm and putting them in a Fallopian tube.
- Egg donation (donor IVF) involves mixing donated eggs from another woman with the partner's sperm, then putting them in the infertile woman's womb.
- Embryo donation – the same can be done with an embryo formed from a donated egg and donated sperm.
- One day it may even be possible to grow a baby in an artificial womb, however unprepossessing a start that might sound!

FOR MEN:
- IUI – intrauterine insemination – placing sperms directly into the womb, usually after hormonal egg stimulation. This makes pregnancy twice as likely.
- IVF (see above).
- ICSI – intracytoplasmic sperm injection – a type of IVF in which an ejaculated or surgically removed sperm is injected directly into a surgically removed egg in a test tube.

- Gondadotrophin therapy.
- Surgical removal of sperm from the testes or epididymis if a man has no sperms in his ejaculated semen.
- Surgery for extensive varicose veins in the scrotum ('varicocele') though recent research suggests this makes little difference.
- Sperm donation (DI – donation insemination) – insemination of a woman with donated sperm.

STORING SPERMS, EMBRYOS AND OVARIAN TISSUE

Men and women who need cancer treatment may risk infertility but they can ask about the possibility of having sperms, embryos or ovarian tissue frozen before treatment begins. Storage techniques are improving all the time and some women have already been successfully impregnated with their partner's sperms saved and stored before his death.

Women may one day be able to decide they want children later in life and have their ovarian tissue, or even embryos, frozen and stored in the meantime. This could be especially useful for young women whose G-Test (see page 12) predicts an early decline in fertility. As I write this, one couple is already planning to have embryos placed in long-term frozen storage so the woman can pursue her career without running the risk of infertility due to her age when she eventually decides she would like a baby.

The complex biological processes that lie behind a woman getting pregnant are amazing whether they happen normally or need a nudge along the way. So now, how about pregnancy itself?

CHAPTER FIVE

Being pregnant

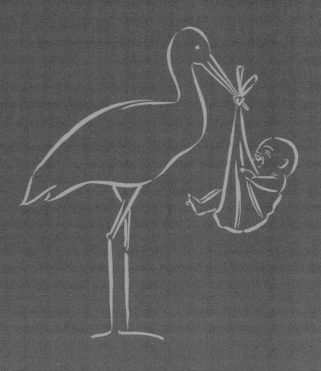

T he waiting time of pregnancy brings its own changes and opportunities. Many women find that being well informed helps them make the most of their new experiences.

HOW YOU'LL KNOW YOU'RE PREGNANT

You may just 'know'. Some women know right from conception. Call it intuition, call it sixth sense, but it happens quite often.

Most women notice some physical changes in the first few weeks. The first is likely to be a missed period. You may feel unusually tired or, from about six weeks after conception, sick in the morning. Your breasts gradually become heavy, full or tender, like before a period. And you may spend a penny more often.

At least three women out of five crave such things as pickles, kippers or chocolate; many even long to eat non-food items such as coal, cement or soil! Others feel extra hungry. And some go off coffee, tea or alcohol, or find food tastes different – perhaps metallic.

Don't be misled into thinking you're not pregnant if you have what you think is a much lighter 'period' than usual. A little bleeding happens fairly often at the time a pregnant woman would otherwise have expected her first one or two periods (see page 93).

You can buy a pregnancy test kit from a pharmacy, or arrange a test with your doctor. Many tests can be used from the day you would have expected your next period. The information leaflet will tell you how accurate the test is likely to be.

WHEN YOU'RE DUE

The average full-term pregnancy – calculated from the first day of the last period – lasts 280 days (40 weeks), though a normal pregnancy may last from 37–42 weeks and only seven per cent of babies arrive on the day they are due.

Work out your 'due' date by marking the first day of your last period on a calendar, going forward nine calendar months, then adding a week.

This form of calculation is in widespread use, though most babies are really a few days younger than it suggests. This is because pregnancy begins at conception (which occurs around ovulation – day 14 in the average cycle) rather than on the first day of the last period!

EMOTIONAL REACTIONS

The day you realise you are pregnant is a day like no other, especially if it's your first baby – and even more so if you've been trying for some time. Emotions such as delight, joy, excitement and awe are there in plenty for the woman who wants to be pregnant, mixed, perhaps, with a tinge of apprehension, anxiety, or even sometimes shock. The older woman, used to years of being child-free, may catch herself wondering, 'Whatever have I done?'

The woman pregnant by mistake may experience shock, disbelief, fear and even anger. Yet there's a good chance that she too may, in time, feel a sense of excitement, pleasure and achievement.

FEELINGS AND CHANGES

Pregnancy offers the chance to change, grow up and mature – and not just physically! Many women gain new insights into themselves and their relationship, feel more deeply and develop a wider perspective on life in general and their own lives in particular. And it means you're about to join a world-wide club.

Men experience similar changes. Like women, many sense a deep commitment to their baby and a welling up of pride and wonder. Yet parenthood is a big responsibility. It helps to discuss his feelings in an open, relaxed way, without criticising or judging, but simply listening, accepting and trying to understand.

It's normal to experience a whole welter of feelings and you may be surprised to find yourself continuing to be particularly emotional throughout pregnancy. Rather as some men claim to think of sex every few minutes, many pregnant women say their thoughts keep returning to their new state and their unborn baby.

If this happens to you, you might forgive your partner for wondering whether you're becoming one-track-minded and, perhaps, for secretly fearing the loss of your attention when the baby arrives. It makes sense to involve him in your progress and plans and sometimes to focus on other things.

YOUR CHANGING BODY AND YOUR BABY'S DEVELOPMENT

Women generally talk about pregnancy as lasting nine calendar months but health care professionals think of it in terms of weeks. This makes the average pregnancy last for ten 4-week months.

First month (weeks 1–4):
You may notice some of the changes mentioned on page 52.

Your baby's life begins when the sperm fertilises the egg – usually in a Fallopian tube; the fertilised egg takes about six days to travel to the womb and burrow into the womb lining, by which time it is a little ball of dividing cells the size of a sugar grain. By the end of the month the embryo is 4mm (under ¼in) long, and the front of the head, the eye sockets and the ears have started to develop.

Second month (weeks 5–8):
The signs of pregnancy become more obvious. Your skin may be dry, flaky or even spotty, and you may sometimes feel faint.

Your baby grows to about 2½cm (1in) long. The organs, arms, legs and face start developing, the heart begins beating and the nervous system is nearly fully developed.

Third month (9–12 weeks):
With luck you'll stop feeling sick. You'll also notice some weight gain and may feel warmer than usual.

Your baby grows to 6½cm (2½in). The bones and external genital organs begin forming, and the fingers, toes and face mature, though the eyes stay closed. By 12 weeks the baby can suck his or her thumb.

Fourth month (13–16 weeks):
You may begin to feel really well – and much less tired – and your tummy may already be swelling.

Your baby grows to 16cm (nearly 7in). The kidneys and other organs are working, finger- and toenails are present, and eyebrows and lashes appear. At 14 weeks the baby may be starting to see, hear, taste, smell and sense touch and pain.

Fifth month (17–20 weeks):
People may say you look 'blooming'. You'll probably feel very well, with thicker, shinier hair and a glowing complexion. You may dream more than usual and some women find their memory isn't as sharp as before.

Your baby grows to 25½cm (10in) and scalp hair begins to grow. You may feel the baby's movements from 18 weeks.

Sixth month (21–24 weeks):
You'll probably feel fine and experience a lot of movement in your womb. Your expanding womb may mean you breathe harder during exercise.

Your baby grows to 33cm (13in) and because the brain cells are maturing fast the baby may react to stimuli such as noise or the warmth of a bath.

Seventh month (25–28 weeks):
You'll almost certainly now have an obvious 'bump' and may feel your womb tightening with occasional 'Braxton Hicks' contractions. These are more obvious versions of the contractions a non-pregnant woman feels during orgasm and, perhaps, at the beginning of a period. They are mini versions of labour contractions. Put your hand on your tummy and you'll feel your womb tightening.

The average baby now weighs almost 1kg (2lb) and can open his or her eyes, suck the thumb and maybe hiccup too. A girl has around 7 million eggs in her ovaries (compare this with later, page 41!) and a boy's scrotum has developed.

Eighth month (29–32 weeks):
Your energy levels will probably fluctuate and you may sometimes feel very tired and have backache. Virtually every woman looks pregnant now.

Your baby goes on growing, weighs about 1½ kg (over 3lb) and can swallow.

Ninth month (33–36 weeks):
You'll really feel the weight of your baby, amniotic fluid, womb, placenta and extra fat.

Your baby could reach nearly 2½ kg (over 5lb) and begin settling into the final birth position.

Tenth month (37–40 weeks):
You'll probably need extra rest.

Your baby grows more – the average birth-weight is 3½–4kg (7½–9lb) at birth.

LOOKING AFTER YOURSELF AND YOUR UNBORN CHILD

Carry on looking after yourself as described in Chapter Three. This seamless pattern of caring for yourself in the months before and after conception is called peri-conceptual care. Its aim is to make you and your baby as healthy as possible and to protect your baby from the earliest moment of life – which is probably well before you realise you are pregnant.

Be a non-smoker. It's more valuable to stop smoking now than at any other time of your life. If you haven't yet stopped, don't forget help is available and successful. But don't use nicotine patches as an aid as they aren't safe in pregnancy. If you really can't stop, opt for middle-tar cigarettes as low-tar varieties cause higher levels of carbon monoxide in the blood and reduce the baby's oxygen supply.

Take special care of your teeth and gums. Gums are softer in pregnancy, which means they are more vulnerable if you neglect regular, efficient tooth cleaning and flossing, and eat a sugary diet. New research suggests that bad gum disease in pregnancy makes it *seven times more likely* that a woman will have a low birth-weight baby. You are entitled to free dental care during pregnancy. However, it's thought safer not to have amalgam fillings either put in or removed during pregnancy.

Don't let yourself get too tired. Ongoing fatigue from overdoing physical or mental work or other activities can, at worst, make pre-term birth and a low-birth-weight baby more likely. One recent study found that working for more than 40 hours a week in a mentally demanding profession makes a woman 40 per cent more likely to have a premature baby.

Turn to Chapters Seven, Eight and Nine for information about eating, drinking, dietary supplements, keeping fit, looking after your figure, relaxing and dealing with common health concerns.

TRAVELLING

Carry any medical information about your pregnancy (such as a 'co-operation card').

When in the car, arrange your seatbelt so the diagonal strap lies between your breasts, and the lower strap beneath your bump.

GOING ABROAD

You may decide to travel only to places where you can rely on medical help in an emergency, especially if any of the following are true:

- You are expecting twins or more.
- You have had a miscarriage or stillbirth before.
- You are getting near your due date.
- Your doctor thinks you are likely to give birth early.

It may make sense to avoid places with a high risk of malaria (East and West Africa, Thailand and Papua New Guinea).

IMMUNISATION

Remind your doctor you are pregnant when discussing travel immunisations. Vaccines containing live viruses (including polio and yellow fever) are unsuitable during pregnancy.

INSURANCE

You may need to pay for extra travel insurance cover.

Take form E111 (available from larger post offices) if travelling within the EC; this entitles you to free or part-free medical care, or allows for reimbursement of some or all costs.

If your destination is remote, make sure your insurance covers

MEDEVAC – a scheme enabling transport to somewhere safe in an emergency.

MEDICAL KIT

Should you need a blood transfusion abroad, check (with embassy staff help if necessary) whether the blood has been screened for HIV and hepatitis infection. If not, the embassy staff may be able to find an expatriate blood donor. Alternatively, you could join the Blood Care Programme before you travel. This undertakes to fly safe blood anywhere in the world with a courier. Details from British Airways Travel Clinics.

Take a sterile medical kit (with needles, syringes and tubes) – available from many large chemists – if travelling outside Western Europe or North America.

FLYING

Most airlines won't accept pregnant travellers after 35 weeks; some refuse after 28.

Don't fly if you are very anaemic or have sickle cell disease, as cabin pressure changes could make you and your baby short of oxygen.

Don't fly if you know your baby has a high risk of being born early.

Don't be concerned about airport security checking devices; they are safe for you and the baby.

Walk around the plane every half-hour, and avoid crossing your legs when seated, as pregnant women have a raised risk of potentially serious blood clots in their leg veins.

WORK – HOW LONG TO CONTINUE

Many women work for as long as they feel fit and well, but it's wise not to make any hard and fast plans as you can't know in advance how you'll feel either before or after your baby is born. One recent study of 16,000 European women concluded that pregnant women should give up their work as long as possible before their baby is due to reduce their risk of miscarriage and premature birth.

TELLING YOUR EMPLOYER

If your job could endanger you or the baby it's best to inform your employer that you're pregnant as soon as possible so your working conditions can be monitored or altered, or your role changed. Potentially hazardous activities include lifting; standing for long periods; working too long, too hard or on shifts; working with ionising 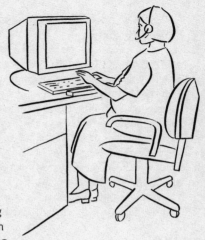 radiation and certain chemicals. You are entitled to alternative work if necessary for your safety.

If you have any questions about employment rights, ring the Maternity Alliance helpline or request their leaflet, *Sickness, Pregnancy and Maternity Leave – Your Employment Rights*.

MATERNITY PAY AND BENEFITS

Information about maternity pay and benefits is available from:

Your employer.

Your benefits agency.

The free leaflet, *Babies and Benefits*, from the Department of Social Security Leaflets Unit, PO Box 21, Stanmore, Middlesex HA7 1AY.

The leaflet, *Pregnant at Work*: send £1 plus an sae to the Maternity Alliance, 45 Beech Street, London EC2P 2LX.

All these try to make the information clear – but it is complicated, so if you don't understand, go on asking until you are satisfied.

Next comes ante-natal care – an important part of being pregnant.

CHAPTER SIX
Ante-natal care

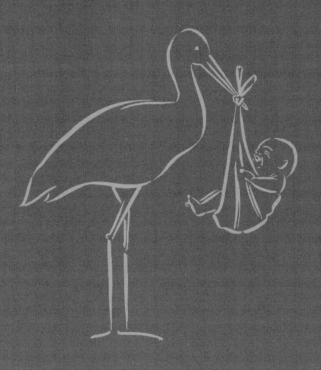

R egular ante-natal care by midwives and doctors helps keep women and their babies safe and healthy and helps identify any problems early.

SEEING YOUR DOCTOR

Make an appointment with your doctor early on. He or she may, with the help of a community midwife, provide most of your ante-natal care, or may ask you to attend hospital more frequently. You are entitled to time off work for ante-natal clinic visits.

At the first visit your doctor will check you are taking a folic acid supplement (see page 28) and aren't on any medication that might harm your baby. You can also discuss where you would like to give birth.

ANTE-NATAL CARE

Your doctor or midwife will check:

- **Your blood pressure**, as high blood pressure may be the first sign of pre-eclampsia (see page 107). It's important to detect this because, at worst, the kidneys stop working properly and the blood pressure spins out of control, allowing protein to leak into the urine, causing fluid retention and putting the woman at grave risk of uncontrollable fits (eclampsia).
- **Your urine for glucose**, a possible though unpredictable sign of diabetes, which appears in up to one woman in ten for the first time in pregnancy. A blood sugar level estimated after a glucose drink is a more accurate test.
- **The growth of your womb and normal growth and development of your baby**. At the first ante-natal visit the staff will weigh you and work out your BMI (body mass index – weight in kilograms divided by height in metres squared). If this is abnormally low, then unless you have good weight gain in the rest of your pregnancy (see page 68), your baby's birth weight may be unhealthily low. You may be weighed at each visit, though some

doctors doubt the value of routine weighing in women with a normal or above average BMI. The doctor or midwife will feel your abdomen and, probably, offer one or more screening tests (such as an ultrasound scan and blood test, see Chapter Eleven) to check whether the baby is growing and developing normally.

- **Your baby's heartbeat**. The midwife or doctor listens to the heart with a small metal trumpet called a fetal stethoscope, or a hand-held ultrasound device.
- **Your blood**, for your group (and Rhesus factor), anaemia, immunity to rubella (German measles), infection (including, perhaps, hepatitis B, syphilis and maybe, soon, H*erpes simplex*) and – if you are of Afro-Caribbean descent – sickle cell disease, or – if of Asian or Mediterranean descent – thalassaemia. If your blood group is Rhesus negative, you will probably be advised to have one or two injections of anti-D immunoglobulin later in pregnancy, to safeguard this and future babies.

YOUR LIKELY SCHEDULE OF VISITS

Traditionally, British women have 15 scheduled ante-natal checks, though several experts suggest as few as eight – or even five – would be just as safe.

Most women have their first hospital check – the so-called 'booking' visit – at around 12 weeks.

ANTE-NATAL CLASSES

Once you are over eight weeks pregnant, enquire about ante-natal classes in your area. Ask your midwife or the hospital ante-natal clinic about NHS classes or consult your local NCT (National Childbirth Trust) teacher about her classes.

Ante-natal teachers provide information about pregnancy and birth. They give expectant women the opportunity for questions and discussion. And they teach relaxation methods – usually muscle relaxation and breathing control – for use in labour.

Most offer a course of several classes, one or all of which is open to expectant fathers too. NHS classes are free, but there is a fee for NCT or other private ones. I think it is worth choosing an 'active birth' class – one whose teacher encourages women to think about moving around during the first stage of labour and change position during the second, so as to make giving birth easier.

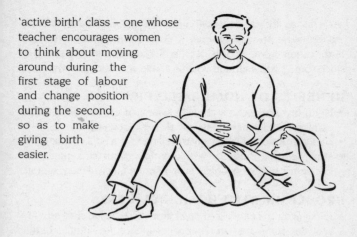

THE MIDWIFE'S ROLE

The midwife is the traditional birth attendant. She (or, very occasionally, he) will look after, encourage and support you, use her skill to facilitate a safe delivery, and call for medical help if necessary.

Many women like to know the midwife who will deliver their baby. The Department of Health's 'Changing Childbirth' policy aims to ensure, first, that every woman knows one of the midwives – her 'named midwife' – involved in her ante-natal care and, second, that at least three out of four women know the person who's to manage their care during delivery.

It's also national policy for more ante-natal care to be managed by midwives with access to doctors, rather than by doctors. A recent survey of 1,299 Glaswegian women found that those managed by midwives were less likely to need their labour induced and less likely to tear or need an episiotomy.

HOME OR HOSPITAL?

About one in 100 women has her baby at home in Britain, and

she's just as likely to do this accidentally, because of a rapid birth, than because she pre-planned it. Some women favour hospital birth, others home, and it can be difficult to decide, especially since some people around you may have very strong views.

BENEFITS OF HOME DELIVERY

- Being on your own patch, with a familiar environment, home comforts, and your nearest and dearest around you.
- No interruption of labour by travelling to hospital to give birth.
- Much less likelihood of well-intentioned but sometimes unnecessary and occasionally even harmful medical intervention.

PROBLEMS WITH HOME DELIVERY

- It's difficult to change midwifery and obstetric facilities so as to provide adequate professional support for home births. Politicians want to fill maternity units, and some medical and nursing staff are reluctant to lose their hospital jobs and work in the community.
- Few family doctors have the experience to be confident and able to deliver women at home these days – though legally they must respond in an emergency.
- Every woman has some risk of serious complications which require urgent medical attention and, perhaps, equipment available only in hospital. For example, serious bleeding after birth is often unpredictable. This occurs in about one woman in 60 and needs skilled help to stop the bleeding and set up a blood transfusion. A baby who doesn't breathe may need skilled medical attention and special equipment – often not available at home. One in 20 women giving birth at home needs to be transferred to hospital for special care.
- The efficient flying squads of trained staff who used to rush to the homes of mothers experiencing these potentially life-threatening problems in labour or afterwards no longer exist. However, the Department of Health intends that all front-line ambulances should be staffed by a paramedic capable of assisting a midwife dealing with an emergency at home.
- Some women live a long way from a maternity unit or doctor, or

in an area where traffic makes rapid travel to hospital in an emergency impossible.

MAKING THE DECISION

You need to weigh up your own feelings and your doctor's advice.

If you want to give birth at home, I suggest you do so only if:

- You live close enough to a maternity unit to be taken there quickly, or close enough to an ambulance station for an ambulance to reach you quickly.
- You can find a doctor willing and able to attend the delivery.
- You can find a midwife comfortable with attending a home birth.
- Your medical history doesn't make this dangerous for you or the baby.

HOSPITAL BIRTHS

Today, almost all women give birth in hospital. They can rest assured that all forward-looking hospital staff want nothing more than for them to enjoy having their babies in a safe, friendly environment.

Many women now go home within 24–48 hours and some hospitals offer the Domino scheme, in which a woman leaves hospital a few hours after having her baby. Some maternity units are run by midwives who call a doctor only if necessary. And some hospitals have labour rooms which are very much more homely than the traditional labour room or ward.

YOUR BIRTH PLAN

You may like to plan how you'd ideally like your labour and birth to be conducted.

Such a birth plan has several functions. Its main one is that it helps you clarify your ideas. It's also a useful discussion document for you and your partner, doctor and midwife. And it guides your birth attendants as to how you think you'd like to be helped and, if necessary, treated.

What a birth plan is *not* is a set of rules, because no one knows

> *What a birth plan is not is a set of rules*

exactly what will happen. This is why it's wise to couch the plan in terms of 'if possible' and 'ideally', and sensible to provide alternatives.

Birth plans arose in the 1970s and 1980s when an explosion of high-tech intervention in labour made the atmosphere surrounding birth very different from what many women wanted. But we now know that even in the most technologically advanced maternity units, willing staff can be sensitive to the wishes of the women they serve. And some take a lot of time and trouble to be so.

HEALTH PROFESSIONALS' ATTITUDES TO OLDER MOTHERS

Older doctors and midwives trained in the 1960s and 1970s were taught about the dangers of being an 'elderly primip' – a woman pregnant for the first time over 35 – and the necessity of treating her like bone china.

But things have changed in the last few decades as improvements in personal and public health, together with advances in technology, have made pregnancy, labour and birth safer for all women. Statistics now show that although older women still have a higher risk of certain problems (see page 21), the risk is in many cases lower than it once was.

Doctors and midwives are particularly concerned if an expectant or labouring woman over 35 is having her first baby and so has no track record of successful pregnancy, labour and birth. This is right and proper, as you deserve the very best care there is.

But however good your professional carers may be, the way you look after yourself is an important part of your personal antenatal care. Top of the list – and the subject of the next chapter – come eating and drinking well.

CHAPTER SEVEN

Eating and drinking

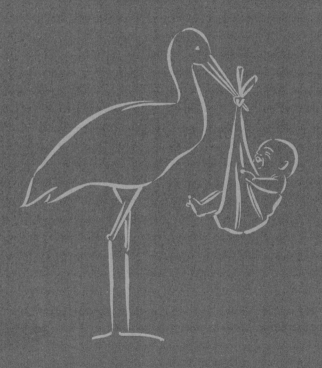

E ating and drinking are among life's greatest pleasures, and a good diet (page 27) in pregnancy helps keep you fit and well and encourages healthy growth and development in your baby.

EXTRA FOOD, AND WEIGHT GAIN

Although you're eating for two, this means one adult and one person who is very small indeed. During the first six months you need no more food than usual. Some women eat less because they feel sick.

From six months on you'll require only a little more food. Experts estimate that the average woman should have around 200 extra calories a day – the amount in a small tomato sandwich!

The average weight gain in pregnancy is 10–12½kg (22–28lb), though some women lose weight and others gain 25kg (55lb) or more. A healthy, balanced diet helps keep your gain within safe, healthy limits. Doctors and midwives are especially concerned nowadays that women should put on *enough* weight (see page 29). So it's just as sensible to eat enough good food as it is not to eat too much 'junk food' – foods laden with saturated fat and refined carbohydrate (white flour and sugar) and low in minerals, vitamins, essential fats and other nutrients, and fibre. A little of this sort of food is fine but too much encourages weight gain and can fill you up so you won't fancy more nutritious fare.

WHICH NUTRIENTS ARE PARTICULARLY IMPORTANT?

During pregnancy folic acid, vitamins B1 and B2 (thiamine and niacin), C and D, and omega-3 fatty acids are particularly important. The nutrients most likely to be lacking in the average diet are folic acid (see page 28 and below), iron, calcium and omega-3s.

Stock up on iron by eating dark-green leafy vegetables, beans and lentils, meat, fish, tofu (soya bean curd), dates, egg yolk, wholegrain foods and fortified breakfast cereals. Orange juice or another good source of vitamin C with meals boosts iron absorption, but avoid tea or coffee with meals as these reduce iron absorption. And leave about an hour before brewing up after a meal. A few women with low iron stores need a daily iron supplement.

Boost your calcium intake with dark-green leafy vegetables (including broccoli), swede, tinned sardines with their bones, soya bean products fortified with calcium, nuts, seeds (including the sesame seed paste, tahini) and dairy food.

Enrich your diet with omega-3s by eating beans and bean products (such as tofu), walnuts and their oil, pumpkin seeds, linseeds, wholegrain-cereal foods, rapeseed oil, meat from grass-fed animals, and a helping a week of oily fish (though see page 27).

VEGETARIANS

Continue to eat a wide variety of foods, making sure you have enough protein (from cheese, milk, yoghurt and other dairy foods; wholegrains – including brown rice; nuts and seeds; peas, lentils and beans – including soya products such as tofu; and Quorn, made from fungal protein).

VEGANS

There's no reason why a pregnant woman and her baby shouldn't be fine on a healthy vegan diet. However, some people who eat a vegan diet go short of vitamin B12. This is most likely if you weren't brought up eating vegan food, because if you've had to teach yourself you may not yet know enough nutritious vegan recipes. Boost your intake with daily helpings of yeast extract (such as Marmite), fortified brewer's yeast, and fortified products such as certain veggie burgers and sausages, breakfast cereals and margarines.

FOODS TO LIMIT OR AVOID

Avoid liver, liver products and vitamin-A-enriched foods as they may contain too much vitamin A to be safe for your baby. Also avoid foods containing raw egg (such as mayonnaise) because getting *Salmonella* gastro-enteritis could harm your baby. See page 38 for tips on which foods to avoid so as to minimise your risk of *Listeria* and *Toxoplasma* infection.

SUPPLEMENTS

Continue with your folic acid supplement (see page 28) for the first 12 weeks. Some US experts suggest continuing throughout pregnancy as a folic acid deficiency raises the risk of low birth-weight.

Doctors no longer routinely recommend iron supplements for all pregnant women as they are necessary for only a few. A routine blood test will show whether you need one.

If you eat poorly it may be worth taking a multi-vitamin and mineral supplement specially formulated for pregnancy (see page 136). Ask your pharmacist for advice on suitable products. If you can't stop smoking, take a vitamin C supplement to replace that lost each time you light up.

If your diet isn't all it could be, then as well as a special multi-vitamin and mineral product, it may be worth taking a supplement of certain essential fatty acids (docosahexaenoic and arachidonic acids, which are omega-3s, and gamma linolenic acid, which is an omega-6 – see page 136) to supply these important nutrients to your baby's developing brain and eyes.

ALCOHOL

Some women stop drinking alcohol completely when pregnant, either because they go off it or because they are worried about it harming their baby (see page 30). But is this necessary?

We know there's a definite association between more than 20 units a week and harm to an unborn baby's developing brain.

Regular drinking of large amounts of alcohol can lead to poor fetal growth, reduced intelligence, a particular facial appearance, and even stillbirth.

Some researchers say there's no evidence of adverse effects on her baby if a pregnant woman drinks 10–15 units a week or less. But others suspect even this is best avoided. US experts, for example, advise pregnant women to abstain completely. However, many UK experts say pregnant women can have no more than one or two units once or twice and week, a unit being a small (83ml or 3fl oz) glass of 12 per cent wine, half-pint (300ml) of 3.5 per cent beer or cider, or a single measure of spirits. Maternal alcohol consumption may be more risky during certain critical stages of fetal brain development.

A possible association between alcohol in pregnancy and leukaemia was reported in 1997. In this US study, 300 women whose babies had leukaemia were three times as likely to have drunk alcohol in late pregnancy than women in a comparison group. Those whose babies had myeloid leukaemia were over ten times as likely to have drunk alcohol!

Evidence also suggests that women who do all these three things – drink a moderate amount of alcohol (more than 12 units a week), drink a lot of coffee (enough to supply over 400mg of caffeine a day, see below) and smoke more than 13 cigarettes a week – have an increased risk of having a low birth-weight baby.

One problem with research is that the size of an alcohol unit isn't the same in each country; it's also difficult to work out how many units there are in an alcoholic drink when the strength of beer and cider, for example, varies so much from one brand to another.

So where does this leave you? Confused, I expect. However, it looks to me as though it's *too much alcohol at any one time* that's most likely to be a problem, not the occasional alcoholic drink. If you want to drink, I suggest you stick to one or, at the absolute most, two units once or twice a week.

COFFEE, TEA AND COLA

A few studies report an association between coffee, pregnancy problems and low birth-weight, but most don't and there's no evidence that moderate amounts are harmful.

However, women's bodies break down caffeine more slowly in pregnancy, especially in the last few months, so if you normally drink a lot of coffee, it's worth cutting down.

The amount researchers deem 'moderate' provides 320–360mg of caffeine a day. One 150ml (6floz) cup of average-strength brew made from ground coffee contains 80–90mg of caffeine; a similar sized, average-strength cup of instant coffee, 60mg.

The average cup of tea or can of cola contains 40mg of caffeine.

MILK

This is an excellent source of calcium and protein but there's no need to drink it if you don't like it, as long as you have a healthy, balanced diet.

FOOD SENSITIVITY

One of the most common food allergies in young children is to peanuts, but researchers disagree as to whether eating them in pregnancy makes a woman's unborn child more likely to develop peanut allergy some time in childhood. However, if you suffer from a food allergy, or have an allergy-prone parent or sibling, it's wise to avoid eating peanuts.

The same applies to other protein foods. In pregnancy you can safely eat anything you like, but it's probably best not to eat lots of it at any one time if there's allergy in your family.

After eating and drinking well, keeping fit is the next most important thing you can do to look after yourself.

CHAPTER EIGHT

Keeping fit

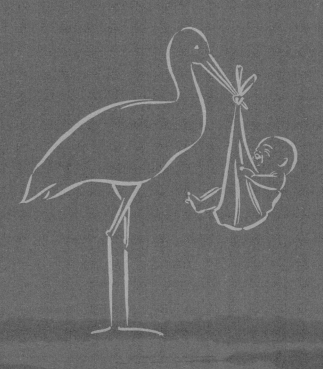

K eeping fit by taking daily exercise is well worthwhile for you – and if you're healthy, your baby benefits too.

BENEFITS OF DAILY EXERCISE

Half an hour's aerobic exercise five days a week, and brisk enough to make you feel warm and get your heart and lungs working harder, will help you keep fit and well. It will help you cope with the weight gain of pregnancy and, hopefully, avoid some common ailments.

Aerobic exercise also helps guard against cardiovascular disease, high blood pressure and non-insulin-dependent diabetes, and produces a natural high by boosting endorphin levels. Being pregnant is no reason to miss out on all this.

Besides aerobic exercise, it's sensible to incorporate some stretching and strengthening exercises into your daily routine. These extend muscles through their whole range of movement and help keep the body strong and supple.

Last but not least are pelvic-floor exercises. Done regularly, these give you more control down below. This helps prevent embarrassing leaks of urine and increases sexual pleasure and, perhaps, gives more sensitive control of how fast the baby's head comes down the vagina in labour.

CHOOSING WHAT'S BEST AND KEEPING IT UP

- The important thing is to choose exercise that's enjoyable and appropriate for you and your stage of pregnancy.
- The best sort of exercise is the one that suits you, your personality and lifestyle and, most important, that you like enough to do! If you aren't sure, consider walking, swimming, cycling, or pregnancy workout classes at your gym or at home with a video and, perhaps, a friend.

- Choose from a range of activities, otherwise daily exercise can be boring.
- Make exercise an essential and important part of the day.
- Adjust your exercise to match your energy level and physical capabilities as the weeks go by.

PRECAUTIONS DURING PREGNANCY

- Check with your doctor before beginning your pregnancy exercise programme if you have had a miscarriage or back trouble.
- Avoid vigorous exercise such as squash or high-impact aerobics if you have had a miscarriage.
- Avoid any exercise that makes you breathless, such as sprinting.
- Tell your instructor you are pregnant.
- You may prefer to avoid risks. Falls, for example, are likely with contact sports, horse-riding or skiing. Your centre of gravity shifts to the front in mid- to late pregnancy, making balancing more difficult. Water-skiing or sliding down a water flume could force water into your vagina. Jumping, scuba diving and high-altitude climbing are potentially hazardous. Jogging jars and may damage loosened joints. And a few sports, such as parachuting, are clearly ill-advised for anyone more than a very few weeks pregnant.

> *A sauna is inadvisable for pregnant women with high blood pressure*

- No one is sure of the effects of short periods of intense heat on babies. A sauna is inadvisable for pregnant women with high blood pressure but if you're healthy, a short period in a sauna would probably do no harm. If you don't want to take any chances, avoid saunas, steam rooms and hot tubs and don't sit in a jacuzzi above 38.5°C.

AND DURING EXERCISE ...

- Wear sports shoes, not slippery socks or tights.
- Start with gentle stretches and warm-up exercises, and cool

down and relax for ten minutes afterwards.

- Don't push yourself to achieve what you did before pregnancy – take advice from a qualified gym or other exercise instructor to adapt your exercise programme if necessary.
- Don't compete.
- Let your body be your guide so you never exercise too hard or too much, or become overheated. Stop if your body tells you you've done enough.
- Stop and contact a doctor or midwife if you bleed or your waters break; or if you have abdominal or chest pain, dizziness, unexpected breathlessness, nausea or vomiting, leg swelling or pain, or headache; or if, after exercise, your baby stops moving as expected.

PELVIC-FLOOR EXERCISES

Your pelvic-floor muscles surround your back passage, vagina and urethra (urine passage). If you aren't sure how to tighten them, start off on the loo with a full bladder. Let some urine go then use your pelvic-floor muscles to stop the stream for four seconds. Repeat several times until your bladder is empty.

Once you have the hang of this and can recognise the muscles involved, you can do it – without passing water – anywhere, any time. All you do is tighten the muscles, hold tight for a count of four, then let go. Repeat five times and do the whole set of exercises several times a day.

PROTECTING YOUR BACK

A pregnancy hormone called relaxin softens ligaments to loosen joints ready for birth. This, plus the increasing weight of your tummy, makes back and joint strain more likely. So protect your back by:

- Keeping a good posture, taking care not to stick your tummy out.
- Making sure that when you lift anything, you bend your knees, not your back.

- Being careful not to strain your lower back while bending or stretching.
- Avoiding breaststroke when swimming, unless you swim with your head well down in the water.
- Not exercising if you have backache – unless you simply stretch out tense back muscles under your instructor's supervision.

THE FIRST THREE MONTHS

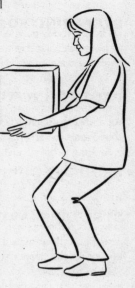

Many women comfortably continue with their usual exercise routine during this time. If you feel sick or otherwise unwell, stop for the time being unless exercise makes you better. Avoid getting too hot during the early months, by wearing the right clothing, having plenty to drink, not overdoing it, and not working out in an overheated place with poor air circulation.

MID-PREGNANCY

Now's the time to think of joining a pregnancy exercise class, using a pregnancy exercise video at home, or consulting a pregnancy exercise book.

Carry on with aerobic exercise, but make sure it's mild to moderate and raises your heart-rate to no more than 140 beats per minute – or a little more if you exercised regularly before pregnancy.

Practise strength and suppleness exercises to help prepare you for an active birth – one in which you move around during the first and second stages of labour (see page 116). The fitter and more supple you are, the easier it will be to get into the positions that make birth easier.

Avoid exercising lying down on your back from now on.

PREPARING FOR LABOUR

Carry on with strength and suppleness exercises, and also with aerobic exercise.

PROTECTING YOUR FIGURE

You can help protect your figure so it's easier to get back into shape after the birth by:
• Wearing a bra at night, and wearing an especially supportive one during exercise.
• Using exercise to keep your muscles toned.

STRETCH MARKS

Stretch marks are scars caused by stretching of the skin during times of great hormonal activity such as pregnancy and puberty. Reduce them by:
• Eating a healthy diet (see pages 27 and 69). Unfortunately this doesn't prevent stretch marks completely since genetic and hormonal factors are involved too.
• Don't overeat, as excess fat stretches skin unnecessarily (though it's good for pregnant women to lay down some extra fat).
• Each day smooth into the skin of your abdomen, hips and thighs either a little oil made by adding two drops each of lavender and neroli oils to a tablespoon of wheatgerm oil, or some aloe vera gel, evening primrose oil or cocoa butter.

Now on to relaxing!

CHAPTER NINE

Relaxing

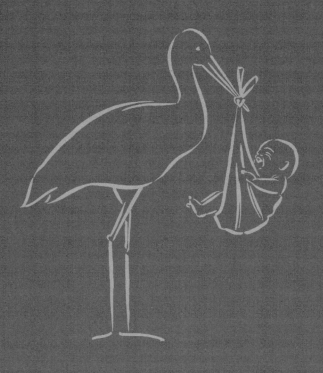

Everyone needs time for rest, relaxation and recreation – and it's especially important if you're expecting your first baby in your 30s or 40s. Why? Because you're probably already fitting a lot into your life and it's unwise to put your – and your baby's – well-being at the bottom of the pile.

Relaxing is one important way of managing stress (see page 82). People relax in different ways. Some like simply doing nothing; others prefer a change of activity, scene or pace, good company, or the unwinding that follows exercise. And many like to be entertained, for example by music, a movie, a book or magazine, or TV.

No one should need an excuse to relax but if you do, there's none better than being pregnant.

SEX, ROMANCE AND SENSUALITY

Sex can be a lovely way to let go the tensions of the day or start the morning. Yet women vary greatly as to whether they feel more – or less – sexy when pregnant, and you may feel differently at various times during your pregnancy.

Men, too, vary, with some fancying their partner even more as her tummy swells. A few are turned off, worried that they'll hurt the baby or their partner, while others feel their partner is now a mother-figure rather than a sex partner. Empathic listening should help both of you air your feelings and, hopefully, let go of any fears and concerns.

However much actual sex you have, make plenty of time for romance – for evenings out and saying how much you love each other – as well as sensual pastimes such as massage with fragrant oils. These help enrich your relationship ready for when the baby comes along.

As your tummy grows, you and your partner will probably be more comfortable with sex in the 'spoons' position (on your sides), or with you on top or on all-fours.

BATHING

Enjoying the luxury of a leisurely, scented, warm bath can be very relaxing and many heavily pregnant women in particular enjoy the sense of weightlessness as the water supports their bodies. The only cautions are not to have your bath too hot, and not to slip when getting out.

MASSAGE

Massage is an age-old aid to relaxing and feeling better. And massaging someone you love is a way of showing that you care for them.

Having a massage in pregnancy can be very soothing. All you need is a warm, draught-free room and some massage oil – sweet almond oil is pleasant. To each tablespoonful of this oil add a few drops of a fragrant essential oil (such as lavender, neroli or ylang-ylang). Certain oils might at very worst encourage miscarriage or damage the fetus, so be sure to avoid:

Arnica, basil, clary sage, hyssop, juniper, marjoram, myrrh, sage and thyme.
Rosemary and sweet fennel (in the first 3–4 months, and after that unless well diluted).
Cypress (until 5 months).
Chamomile and lavender (if you have ever miscarried).
Rosemary (if you have high blood pressure).

Details of where to buy high-quality essential oils and an aromatherapy massage oil specially blended for pregnant women are on page 136.

EATING

Many women relax by taking time to cook creatively. This brings a double bonus during pregnancy, when a nutritious diet is so important.

STRESS MANAGEMENT

We all develop ways of managing and relieving stress. Even though our chosen methods at any one time may not be the best, they are often the best we can choose at the time. But as time passes, we may realise that our favourites cause more problems than they prevent or cure. And it's then that many of us decide to find better ways.

Smoking, drinking too much alcohol and comfort-eating are common stress-relievers but are potentially harmful to men's and women's fertility (see Chapter Four) and may affect the baby during pregnancy. This is why it's wise to replace them with other, non-damaging alternatives (see below).

SMOKING

Researchers report that 14 per cent of women who smoke when pregnant say they find it relaxing, 32 per cent say it relieves stress, 14 per cent do it when bored, and 22 per cent enjoy it. Yet the researchers suggest these women are either denying the risks of smoking to their babies (let alone to themselves), or playing down their importance.

Smoking during pregnancy makes a miscarriage more likely. It can also damage your baby's health, raise the risk of low birth-weight, and make your new-born more likely to have health problems such as asthma or even to die from a cot death. As a means of relaxation, it simply isn't worth the risk.

Becoming a non-smoker means finding other ways of relaxing, other strategies for relieving stress (see below) or boredom, and other sources of pleasure. This can be done. But it takes determination, courage, persistence and the awareness of how best to do it. It may also take the courage or humility to accept help and support.

Here are some tips:

- Decide on a day to become a non-smoker.
- Suggest that your partner – or someone else – stops with you.
- Find other rewards, treats or stress-relievers.
- Arrange for company and support when the going gets tough.
- Keep busy at these times.
- Keep reminding yourself why it matters.
- Save the extra cash for a treat or something for the baby.
- Avoid smokers and smoky places.
- Ask for help if necessary.
- Contact a quit-smoking organisation or group (see page 135) for more suggestions and for support.
- Passive smoking is unwise too as it makes both a pre-term birth and a low birth-weight baby more likely. So encourage any smokers with whom you live or work to give up and, in the meantime, try to avoid being in smoke-filled places.

> *Smoking during pregnancy makes a miscarriage more likely*

ALCOHOL

If you do decide to drink alcohol when you're pregnant (see page 70), make it only the occasional glass – or go for a spritzer (half wine, half water), shandy (half beer, half lemonade or ginger beer), or other low-alcohol drinks.

For help with problem drinking, contact Alcoholics Anonymous (see your local phone directory).

COMFORT-EATING

Many people turn to food – and usually to fatty, stodgy food, though any will do – when they are stressed. If you do, and therefore either aren't eating a healthy diet or are overeating and lugging around unnecessary fat as well as the growing weight of your womb, you need to find other stress relievers (see below).

RECREATIONAL DRUGS

Learn to say 'no'. For the sake of your child's health and well-being these powerful substances have no place before, during or after pregnancy. You may need to learn effective assertion skills so you can say no to drugs from friends or pushers. One part of being assertive is finding healthy ways of boosting your self-confidence and self-esteem.

EFFECTIVE STRESS MANAGEMENT

The good news is that many women in their 30s and 40s already know how to handle stress effectively.

If you'd like to know more, here's a four-point plan:

1. **Recognise when things are getting too much**. For example, you may feel anxious, with shallow breathing and a tension headache, or be snappy, exhausted or miserable. Continued stress symptoms aren't good for your health or fertility, and may not be good for your baby either.

2. **Identify who or what makes you stressed** – then, if possible, either remove the stressor or modify it.

3. **Practise effective stress-relieving strategies**. The list of possibilities is huge and the following examples are gleaned from many people:

   Lifestyle: Eat a healthy diet; choose calming foods – for example, high-carbohydrate, high-fibre, low-protein snacks such as a banana, a wholemeal salad sandwich or a baked potato; create a more relaxed eating style; reduce your caffeine intake; aim for enough good quality sleep; take regular aerobic exercise.

   Relaxation: Practise immediate relaxation techniques – such as breathing exercises and whole body relaxation; have some time off; enjoy a sybaritic bath; organise breaks, outings and holidays; enjoy hobbies and other recreational interests; spoil yourself; laugh; cry; find new interests; make time to play; appreciate – perhaps at the end of each day – the enjoyable things you've done; make time for contemplation, meditation or prayer.

Environment: Make your surroundings more pleasant, get rid of physical stressors such as a poor chair.

Balance and perspective: Recognise what really matters; challenge 'shoulds, oughts and musts'; forgive yourself; see stressful situations as opportunities; accept the inevitable; tolerate situations in which you can't make clear choices; avoid perfectionism; sift information to avoid overload; recognise negative thinking and behaviour, decide whether these are worthwhile and give them up if not; adopt realistic expectations; learn from mistakes; separate thoughts from feelings; put problems in perspective without blowing them up or belittling them; dwell on positives; don't jump to conclusions.

Outside help: Offload on family and friends; ask for counselling or medical help; use alternative therapies; arrange financial advice.

Self management: Listen to your mind and body; be assertive – not passive or aggressive; accept yourself for who you are, only criticising your behaviour if necessary; recognise your good points; practise problem-solving techniques; practise – in your mind's eye – new ways of behaving; encourage and affirm yourself; learn to make decisions.

Time management: Prioritise, set realistic deadlines, do important tasks when you feel freshest, anticipate and plan for

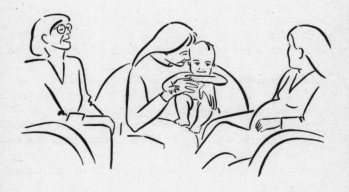

stressful times; make time for yourself each day; don't do too much; learn to say 'no'.

Relationships: Nurture and enjoy intimate relationships; keep in touch with friends; deal with relationship problems; encourage and affirm those around you; recognise the feelings of others, and separate them from your own; delegate.

4. **Take steps to give up unhelpful stress-relievers**, such as smoking, or drinking or eating too much (see above).

Help with stress is available from books, stress-management trainers, counsellors and MIND (Granta House, 15–19 Broadway, Stratford, London E15 4BQ, tel: 020 8522 1725).

You may find that effective, safe stress-relieving strategies help when dealing with common concerns in pregnancy.

CHAPTER TEN

Common concerns

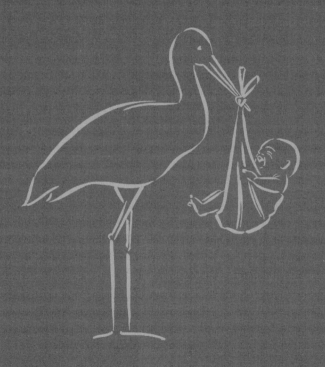

L ife wouldn't be life without problems, and pregnancy is no exception to the rule. The good news is that information gleaned from other women's experiences, together with years of scientific research, can be a real help.

FATIGUE

Pregnant women of any age often feel tired in the first three months, then much perkier – possibly even less tired than usual – in the middle three and, finally, increasingly easily fatigued in the last three months.

Different people have different energy levels, and whether or not your energy flags during pregnancy probably depends as much on your health, *joie de vivre* and activity and stress levels as it does on your age. However, it's likely (though unprovable) that some women pregnant for the first time in their 30s and 40s feel more tired than they would have done 10, or 20 or more years before.

Deal with fatigue by looking after yourself (see page 56), reducing stress (see page 82) and putting your feet up when necessary. There are no prizes for overdoing things.

FEELING SICK

Nausea – even vomiting – occurs in eight out of ten pregnant women. It's related to high levels of the hormone chorionic gonadotrophin and can occur at any time of the day or night. There are, however, two rays of light here. First, it usually improves from 12 weeks – though this doesn't help the small group of women .who continue to suffer. And, second, it's less common in older women.

Some women find nothing helps except time. However, although the sickness won't harm your baby, it's very unpleasant for you, so try:

- A little carbohydrate, such as dry bread, before getting up.
- Sips of water or carbonated (fizzy) drink.
- Avoiding fried or other fatty foods.
- Avoiding car, bus or boat travel.
- Resting more and not getting over-tired.
- Small, frequent meals.
- Avoiding bitter foods and drinks (such as coffee, lettuce, Brussels sprouts).
- Chewing fresh ginger root or ginger gum (from pharmacies), or drinking ginger root tea.
- Applying light pressure to acupressure point PC-6 (three finger-widths above the crease on the front of the wrist, between the two tendons in the centre) for ten minutes four times a day, or wearing an elastic wrist band sold for sea-sickness (see page 136).
- Remedies made from tamarind or chamomile from a medical herbalist.
- A multi-vitamin and mineral supplement specially formulated for pregnancy (see page 136).

> *Nausea – even vomiting – occurs in eight out of ten pregnant women. It's less common in older women*

If necessary, see your doctor.

HEARTBURN

Heartburn is triggered by the top of the growing womb pushing up against your stomach and encouraging stomach contents to backflow up the gullet. These tips may help:
- Don't eat or drink too much at any one time.
- Eat a healthy diet.
- Have small, frequent meals rather than fewer, large ones.
- Eat slowly and relax at mealtimes.
- Drink fluids only between meals.
- Have an extra pillow or two in bed, or prop up the head of the bed with books under the legs.

- Keep off alcohol and rich foods containing saturated fats and refined carbohydrates (such as pastry, and many desserts, cakes and biscuits).
- Allow several hours between your last main meal and bedtime.
- Avoid excessive weight gain.
- Ask your doctor or pharmacist to recommend an antacid, or a 'rafting agent' such as an alginate.

CRAMP

Why cramp is more common in the last few months of pregnancy isn't clear, but possible remedies include:
- Daily aerobic exercise.
- Warm-up and cool-down periods before and after exercise.
- A healthy diet.
- More dietary magnesium from foods such as wholegrain foods, nuts, soya beans, milk, fish and meat.
- A warm bath before bedtime
- Enough warmth in bed.
- Firm massage.
- And, strange but true, a cork or a magnet beneath the foot of the mattress.

VARICOSE VEINS AND PILES

Pregnancy hormones and pressure from your growing womb may make some of your leg veins varicose (unduly large and even knobbly). Try:
- Having a daily half-hour of aerobic exercise.
- Avoiding standing for long periods.
- Keeping your legs uncrossed when seated.
- Resting with your legs above the level of your abdomen.
- Wearing support tights.
- Eating a healthy diet with plenty of foods rich in vitamin C and flavonoids (especially berries such as blueberries).
- You may also suffer from piles, which are varicose veins around the back passage. If so, check that you are drinking enough and

eating enough high-fibre foods to keep your bowel motions soft and easy to pass without straining.

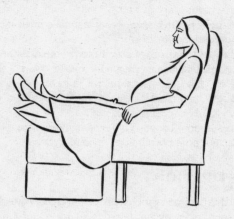

BACKACHE

Take care of your back (see page 76), making sure you keep fit so its muscles are strong. Regular stretching exercises, and maintaining a good posture also help. Massage may ease backache by helping tense muscles relax. If necessary, try taking paracetamol, but don't take aspirin, ibuprofen or other non-steroidal anti-inflammatory painkillers, as experts recommend avoiding these in pregnancy.

Extra bed rest often makes backache worse, so take daytime rests in a chair with your legs up.

When you go to bed, try one of these three tips:
1. Lie on your side with a pillow between your knees.
2. Lie on your side with your upper leg bent at the knee and with that knee pushed slightly forwards and resting on a pillow.
3. If you sleep on your back, put a pillow or two beneath your slightly bent knees.

If all else fails, consult an obstetric physiotherapist, registered osteopath or chiropractor.

CARPAL TUNNEL SYNDROME

The carpal tunnel syndrome – tingling and numbness in the third, fourth and fifth fingers – is generally caused in pregnancy by fluid retention. This waterlogging leads to pressure on the nerve supplying these fingers as it passes through the wrist. The condition will disappear soon after you have given birth.

If you find that tingling and numbness come on after lying in bed with your arm dangling out of the side and your wrist bent, wear a wrist splint at night.

If it comes on after you've been working at a keyboard, rest your wrists on a support in front of your keyboard.

CONSTIPATION

Counter this common problem, experienced by one in two pregnant women, by drinking plenty of fluids, eating a healthy diet with plenty of fibre (salads, vegetables – especially beetroot – fruit and wholegrain foods) and taking exercise.

Some types of iron tablet cause constipation, so if your doctor has recommended them, ask for an alternative mild laxative, such as bran, ispaghula husk, sterculia, methylcellulose or lactulose.

Don't take laxatives without consulting your doctor.

ITCHING

Ease the itching of dry skin by applying moisturising cream mixed with a few drops of lavender oil, and put some bicarbonate of soda into your bath water – but don't soak for too long.

If the itching seems to come from inside, there's little you can do other than take your mind off it. See your doctor if it continues for more than a few days, and especially if your skin has a yellow tinge because, very rarely, itching is caused by one of several liver problems such as intrahepatic cholestasis of pregnancy (ICP). Although a woman with ICP returns to normal after the birth, there's a risk to the baby, so doctors like to monitor such a pregnancy closely and may have to induce labour early.

THRUSH AND BACTERIAL VAGINOSIS

The vaginal and vulval itching and discharge of thrush is caused by infection with the yeast *Candida albicans*. You can treat it with anti-fungal cream and pessaries bought over the counter – ask your pharmacist or doctor for more information.

It's important not to mistake another infection, bacterial vaginosis, for thrush, because the treatments are different. Also, some doctors suspect that untreated bacterial vaginosis (which is present in one pregnant woman in five) is a major trigger of pre-term labour (see page 103). So if your symptoms don't clear up with thrush treatment, or you aren't sure what's wrong, consult your doctor. Bacterial vaginosis is treated with antibiotics (such as oral metronidazole or topical clindamycin).

URINE LEAKS

- Do pelvic-floor exercises several times a day (see page 76).
- Wear an absorbent, waterproof-backed pad.
- Don't let your bladder overfill.
- Avoid the sort of physical exertion or movement that triggers a leak.

BLEEDING

A little vaginal 'breakthrough' bleeding occurs in one in ten pregnancies that continue perfectly normally (see page 52) so the odds are that it's quite harmless.

However, continued bleeding, perhaps with abdominal pain, is one of the first signs of miscarriage. It can also be a sign of other problems, including an ectopic pregnancy (see page 107), something amiss with the cervix or vagina or, rarely, a blood disorder.

WHAT TO DO

- Call an ambulance or contact your nearest maternity unit without delay if you bleed very heavily or feel faint. Later in pregnancy bleeding can be a sign of *placenta praevia* (see page 101), in which case a Caesarean operation may be needed to save your baby's life.

- Call your doctor if you are spotting or bleeding lightly. Your doctor may arrange an ultrasound scan within a few days if you are bleeding lightly, or the same day if the bleeding is heavy. This indicates whether your baby is still alive; if so, you have a nine out of ten chance that all will be well. If there's any uncertainty, you may need another scan 7–10 days later. Even if you stop bleeding, your doctor may recommend a scan to make sure the baby is all right.

- Your doctor should check your blood group and, if it's Rhesus-negative, may give you an injection of anti-D immunoglobuin to prevent rhesus incompatibility in a future pregnancy with a Rhesus-positive baby. This may not be necessary if your bleeding stops by 12 weeks.

- In over 95 per cent of women who bleed, the baby's survival is determined before bleeding begins; nothing you do makes any difference. However, it's sensible to avoid penetrative sex and not to have an orgasm until a day or two after the bleeding stops.

- Don't use tampons.

- And if your work is physically onerous, have a few days off. However, there is no evidence that rest in itself influences the outcome of a threatened miscarriage.

- Finally, continue to care for yourself as recommended in Chapter Three, being careful not to lift heavy weights or stand for long periods of time.

MISCARRIAGES

Unfortunately, you're more likely to miscarry if you're older. Half of all 40-year-old pregnant women miscarry, compared with one in three women overall. Up to two in five miscarriages remain unexplained. Of the remainder, the commonest trigger is a damaged or genetically abnormal baby. Other possible reasons include an immune problem (such as antiphospholipid antibody formation – see page 96, and pre-eclampsia). Or there could be a reaction against the placenta, a low folic acid intake, infection (flu and other viral infections, Listeria and Toxoplasma – see page 38 – Chlamydia, and bacterial vaginosis), disease (such as poorly controlled diabetes or a liver disorder caused by pregnancy – ICP, see page 92), excessive alcohol or smoking, environmental and occupational hazards (see pages 36 and 46), a hormone imbalance (for example, polycystic ovary syndrome, see page 48), a mis-shapen womb, a weak cervix, or fatigue (see pages 56 and 88). It has also been suggested that stress may play a part.

Up to two in five miscarriages remain unexplained

HOW DO YOU KNOW YOU ARE MISCARRYING?
• You may have low tummy-ache, like period pain.
• You will experience bleeding, which will change in colour from dark red to bright red.
• The bleeding continues until the baby, placenta and membranes all come away. In the first month this may be like a period or, possibly, a little heavier. The more advanced your pregnancy, the heavier the bleeding.
• After the first month you may see a small but heartbreakingly recognisable baby.

WHAT HAPPENS THEN?
• Your blood loss will probably dry up over the next week or so.
• If you continue to bleed, your doctor may recommend an 'evacuation' – an operation to remove any remnants of the pregnancy which might otherwise become infected or cause continued bleeding. If you are bleeding heavily you may need to have this done at once.
• Be gentle with yourself; remember that your partner has lost his baby too; and allow yourselves time to grieve.

REPEATED MISCARRIAGE
Some women experience the misery of repeated miscarriage. Officially this means three or more miscarriages. Tests and other

investigations aren't generally offered until then.

However, if you feel time is running out, ask your doctor for blood tests and an ovary scan after just one miscarriage.

A simple blood test can detect antiphospholipid (Hughes) syndrome – in which antiphospholipid antibodies cause multiple small blood clots in the placenta. This condition is more common in women with lupus (an auto-immune disorder causing a variety of possible health problems). If a woman has antiphospholipid syndrome, then taking a small daily dose of aspirin (and, possibly, heparin – an anticoagulant drug), turns her previously very high chance of a further miscarriage into a high chance of a successful pregnancy.

Ultrasound scans reveal that four out of five women who miscarry repeatedly have multiple cysts on their ovaries (polycystic ovaries). If these women are also overweight, then weight loss before the next pregnancy helps prevent another miscarriage (see page 29).

There's a 50:50 chance that investigations won't reveal a cause, but it's certainly worth trying. The advice in Chapters Three and Four may help reduce your risk of another miscarriage, as may aerobic exercise (see page 30).

TAKE SPECIAL CARE OF YOURSELF

If you are in your 30s or 40s and were expecting your first baby you may be particularly upset if you miscarry. Perhaps:

You waited a long time before deciding to get pregnant and now have to wait even longer until you become pregnant again.

You've had one or more miscarriages before.

You became pregnant after trying unsuccessfully for some time.

You've spent a lot of time, energy, money and emotion on assisted conception.

You're used to making successful plans but this one has gone very wrong.

You'll need to take special care of yourself at this disappointing time. Having a break before becoming pregnant allows you to mourn and to separate this lost baby emotionally from the next one you may have. It also gives your body time to restore regular menstrual cycles, so making it easier to work out when you conceive next time. This is worthwhile even though waiting may seem unattractive if you're in your 30s or 40s and feel that time is running out.

A common concern of many older pregnant women is whether or not to have screening and other special tests. We'll look at these in the next chapter.

CHAPTER ELEVEN

Special tests

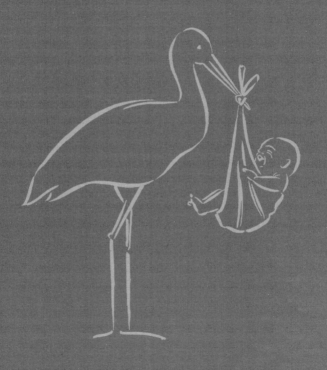

Women expecting their first baby in their 30s and 40s have, on balance, more tests during pregnancy. And they may be more anxious about them than younger women.

WHY MIGHT I BE OFFERED SPECIAL TESTS, AND WHAT ARE THEY?

With the exception of ultrasound scans, which can also be useful in detecting or tracking the progress of pregnancy, screening tests are offered to detect structural malformations and other genetic abnormalities in a baby. Most of these are caused wholly or partly by genetic variation, with Down's syndrome and spina bifida being the best known.

Overall, one or two women in every 100 gives birth to a baby with a malformation. Older mothers have a relatively higher risk.

Doctors offer screening tests as early as possible so that if a subsequent, more accurate test then reveals an abnormality, a couple can have the choice of an abortion. However, *there is no necessity – nor should there be any medical pressure – to have your baby investigated for abnormality, even if your age makes this more likely*. The choice is yours.

If you want to know more about the purpose, accuracy, side-effects and implications of a test or procedure so you can make an informed decision about whether to have it – or if you are upset about anything – go no further until you have discussed your concerns with your medical adviser or midwife.

Screening tests currently on offer to some, or all, women include ultrasound scans (for fetal size and development); blood tests (for the risk of genetic abnormality, or for HIV screening); and the fetal fibronectin test (to assess the risk of prematurity).

A high-risk, or 'positive', screening test result means you'll be offered a further procedure which allows a more accurate test to be done. If this test shows that your baby is definitely abnormal, your doctor will offer you an abortion.

The definition of 'high-risk' varies, but generally a risk of one or more in 250 of a baby being affected is considered high or 'positive'. This also, of course, means there's a 249 chance in 250 that the baby is *not* affected.

Procedures allowing accurate tests for chromosomal abnormalities include: amniocentesis (amniotic fluid sampling) with fetal cell chromosome culture; chorionic villus sampling (placenta sampling) with chromosome culture; and fetal blood sampling (cordocentesis) with chromosome culture.

These procedures are described as 'invasive' because they carry a risk to the baby.

ULTRASOUND SCANNING

In the UK 95 per cent of women have one or more scans in pregnancy. During a scan a technician slides a probe – which emits high-frequency sound waves – over the skin of your abdomen. Reflected sound bounces back from the baby and is picked up and electronically transformed into a screen image. Sometimes the probe is placed in the vagina to give a clearer image (to show, for example, whether a woman has miscarried early in pregnancy). Your baby may move around more during a scan.

Most doctors believe scans are safe for babies and claim that even if any risk were proven, the advantages would far outweigh it.
A scan at 10–14 weeks Confirms whether your baby's size matches your dates, and picks up about 70 per cent of major structural abnormalities (including anencephaly and spina bifida). A neck – or 'nuchal' – scan can, along with the mother's age, predict the risk of Down's syndrome. Early scanning allows earlier risk-prediction of Down's syndrome than does serum screening (see below) and also detects multiple pregnancy.
A scan at 18–20 weeks This will pick up most structural malformations and gives information about the growth and development of the placenta, skull, spine and major organs.
A scan at other times This will be to check whether:
The baby has been miscarried (see page 94).
The pregnancy is ectopic (see page 107).
The cervix is working competently.

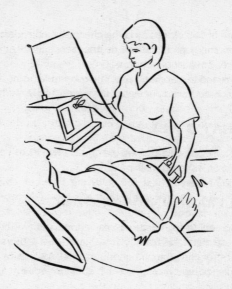

There's a *placenta praevia* – a placenta lying dangerously low in the womb.

The baby is mature enough to be born.

The baby is lying in a good position.

MATERNAL SERUM SCREENING

Serum screening for Down's syndrome (and other major chromosomal abnormalities) is offered by many hospitals between 15 and 20 weeks; an ultrasound scan first confirms the baby's age. Serum screening detects up to three or four Down's babies out of five and is most accurate in older women. It can also indicate a high risk of spina bifida. However, false positives and negatives are possible.

The double, triple and quadruple tests measure the

> *Serum screening detects up to three or four Down's babies out of five and is most accurate in older women*

levels of two, three or four biochemical markers (alpha-fetoprotein, chorionic gonadotrophin, oestriol and inhibin A) in the mother's blood. The risk of abnormality is estimated by looking at both the result and the woman's age. The quadruple test is the most reliable and detects seven or eight out of every ten Down's babies.

WHAT'S NEW?

- A DIY urine test to assess the likelihood of your baby having Down's syndrome is on its way.
- Some researchers are studying whether tests of a baby's genetic material in the mother's blood – present in four pregnancies out of five – should replace amniocentesis when screening for chromosomal abnormalities; they think such a test might be reliable from 11 weeks. Others are studying a test of HCG (human chorionic gonadotrophin) and pregnancy-associated protein A, which could be done at 10–14 weeks.

CHORIONIC VILLUS SAMPLING (CVS)

Sampling and testing cells taken from the placenta is offered at 11–12 weeks. Guided by ultrasound scanning, the doctor puts a needle through the woman's abdominal wall into the placenta and sucks out some cells. Chromosomes are then karyotyped ('cultured', or grown) then examined for genetic problems. The result is available in 1–2 weeks. Sometimes repeat testing is necessary.

The sampling is occasionally done through the cervix.

One or two babies in 100 are miscarried after CVS. Experts are as yet unsure whether this procedure can cause finger, toe and limb deformities. However, even if studies prove this is possible, the risk to any one baby is likely to be small.

AMNIOCENTESIS

Amniocentesis is offered from 14–18 weeks to women with a high risk of an abnormal baby.

The doctor takes a sample of amniotic fluid from around the baby through a needle passed through the wall of the woman's abdomen and into the womb under the guidance of a real-time ultrasound scan. Chromosomes from the baby's cells in the fluid are then karyotyped ('cultured', or grown) and examined for genetic problems. The result is available within three weeks.

Your obstetrician will probably recommend amniocentesis if you have a family history of genetic abnormalities, or if your serum screening suggests a high risk. However, the beguilingly nicknamed 'amnio' isn't always as straightforward as it may sound:

The needle occasionally damages a baby.

At least one in every 100 babies dies afterwards.

Chromosomes fail to grow about three times in 1,000.

FETAL BLOOD SAMPLING (CORDOCEN-TESIS)

After 18 weeks an unborn baby's blood can be sampled if there's any risk of a potentially dangerous infection, for example with rubella or toxoplasmosis. Guided by a real-time ultrasound scan the doctor passes a needle through the wall of the woman's abdomen into her womb and then into the baby's umbilical vein.

The procedure kills one or two in every 100 babies.

TESTS FOR FETAL FIBRONECTIN AND BACTERIAL VAGINOSIS

The new fetal fibronectin test – currently still under evaluation by researchers – indicates whether pre-term labour is likely. It can be done in women who might be at risk because, for example, of early contractions, hydramnios (excess fluid in the womb), a previous premature labour, or twins. Swabs of vaginal mucus taken in weeks 24–27 are tested for a protein called fetal fibronectin. If present after 20 weeks this indicates a strong (one in five) chance of pre-term labour occurring within the next four weeks. These vaginal swabs are also tested for an infection called bacterial vaginosis (see pages 39 and 93) which can encourage the membranes to break down, so raising the fibronectin level and encouraging pre-term birth.

FETAL KICK CHART

If there's reason to be concerned about your baby, your doctor may ask you to record how often the baby moves. In the last few months of pregnancy there are generally at least ten kicks in a 12-hour period.

OTHER HORMONE TESTS

Measurement of the amount of oestriol or placental lactogen produced by the placenta indicates how well this organ is performing. This may be done if your baby seems too small for the duration of pregnancy, or if labour seems to be overdue.

DECIDING ABOUT ABORTION IF YOUR BABY IS ABNORMAL

This decision involves personal, social, moral, spiritual and medical issues and the process – and the action, if you take it – is a life event you'll never forget. While some women find the decision easy, others say it's the hardest thing they've ever done. You may feel under pressure to have a 'perfect' baby. And with so much emphasis from doctors on searching for abnormality and, by implication, on the negativity of having an abnormal child, the reality of discovering you are carrying a less than perfect baby could make you so anxious and afraid that you plunge headlong into the decision to abort.

Several things could help put the issue into perspective:
- Knowing more about the long-term implications of bringing up a child with the problem in question.
- Looking at your 'imperfect' baby as one human being to another. Bringing up a Down's child, for example, isn't always

easy – but the same is true for any child. There's no evidence to show that Down's children have a more negative experience of life than others. And many parents report great rewards from their Down's child.

- A few people – interested in the fact that the extra chromosome in each Down's child's cell profoundly alters anti-oxidant levels – suggest this may cause the physical and intellectual problems they face. They believe these problems could therefore be potentially preventable – even correctable – by therapy with mineral, vitamin, amino acid and other nutritional supplements. This revolutionary idea is completely unproven scientifically, and it would be unwise to build false hopes – but it's very interesting and proper research is in the pipeline.

SHOULD YOU BE SCREENED EVEN IF YOU THINK YOU'D NEVER HAVE AN ABORTION?

Many doctors suggest that such tests are worthwhile even for the woman who disagrees with abortion, because knowing her baby has an abnormality gives her and her partner time to become used to the idea and prepare to welcome their baby. However, I think some doctors really believe that a woman may well change her mind about an abortion once she is confronted with the reality of carrying an abnormal baby.

GENETIC COUNSELLING

Genetic counselling can help you decide whether specific tests are advisable if you have a family history of genetic disorders. Your doctor will tell you where it's available.

For most women tests show they are highly likely to be carrying a normal, healthy baby. But whether or not this is so, certain special situations can occur.

CHAPTER TWELVE

Special situations

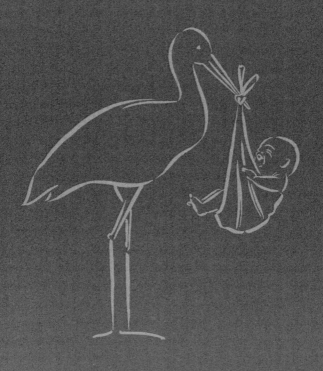

C ertain special situations are either more common during pregnancy in older women or have special significance for them.

ECTOPIC PREGNANCY

One in 100 pregnancies is ectopic, meaning the baby develops outside the womb, usually in a Fallopian tube. Such pregnancies hardly ever produce live babies. An ectopic pregnancy causes bleeding, pain and shock in the woman and is life-threatening, making emergency treatment a necessity.

Ectopic pregnancy is more common in the over-35s, possibly because their Fallopian tubes no longer waft eggs or embryos along to the womb quickly enough for implantation to occur in the proper place. Tubal surgery and assisted conception for previous infertility problems make an ectopic more likely, as does previous use of the progestogen-only Pill or an intra-uterine contraceptive device (see page 32).

Once you've had an ectopic you have an increased risk of it happening again, so you'll probably be offered an ultrasound scan at six weeks next time. If you do have another ectopic, you can then have surgery early. It's also worth having a test for *Chlamydia* infection because when present in the pelvis this makes ectopic pregnancy more likely.

PREGNANCY-INDUCED HYPERTENSION AND PRE-ECLAMPSIA

High blood pressure in pregnancy, with or without a significant leakage of protein into the urine (when the condition is known as pre-eclampsia, as it heralds the possibility of the dangerous fits of eclampsia), is more common in older women, especially those over 36. Regular ante-natal care allows early detection and treatment of raised blood pressure. The baby's birth can then be induced early if necessary.

The following may protect you against high blood pressure in pregnancy (though all except good nutrition are unproven):

- Good nutrition.
- A sexual relationship with the baby's father which continued for at least a year before conception and didn't involve a condom or diaphragm. Interestingly, this allows a woman to develop immunity to her partner's sperm and this is thought to protect her from developing high blood pressure triggered by sensitivity to his sperms!
- A multi-vitamin and mineral supplement specially formulated for pregnancy.
- Daily aspirin may be recommended for some women with early pre-eclampsia.
- Avoiding intense heat, such as in a sauna.

INFECTIONS

Any serious viral infection in early pregnancy readily causes miscarriage.

Flu. Late in pregnancy flu can, at worst, cause stillbirth. If you get a bad attack of flu, anti-viral drug treatment is not suitable during pregnancy, so all you can do is look after yourself and hope all will be well.

Rubella (German measles). If you get rubella in the first 8–10 weeks your baby has a high (90 per cent) risk of getting it and being seriously damaged. By 16 weeks the risk has fallen to 10–20 per cent; after that damage is rare.

So if you are exposed to rubella, then whether or not you've been immunised or had rubella in the past, ask your doctor for an injection of immunoglobulin antibodies. This should reduce the severity of your symptoms and may mean your baby has a reduced risk of damage.

At the same time your doctor will take some blood to be tested for evidence of the infection. You may need another test later. If you become infected, you can hope for the best or ask for an abortion.

Herpes. Genital infection with *Herpes simplex* virus in the last few months of pregnancy raises the risk of a pre-term baby. And it's more likely than an infection earlier in pregnancy to infect the baby during birth and give him or her a potentially dangerous Herpes infection.

Tell your doctor if you have symptoms of genital Herpes (itching, soreness, small blisters or ulcers which burn when you pass urine, swollen lymph nodes in the groin, and perhaps a headache and fever) so you can be treated early.

Chickenpox. Chickenpox can be more serious for women in pregnancy. In the first three months it gives a one in 100 chance of miscarrying, and from 13–20 weeks a one in 50 chance. In the first three months of pregnancy it can also cause limb or other defects in the baby. Later it isn't as serious but can give the baby shingles and hamper growth. If you get chickenpox in the week before or after giving birth, your baby risks having a serious or even fatal infection.

This is why, if you've been in contact with chickenpox, your doctor will arrange a blood test to see if you have any immunity to the infection. If you haven't, an injection of specific immunoglobulin antibodies will make a severe attack much less likely and so help protect your baby. Don't worry about having to wait for the test result before having the antibody injection; waiting for up to ten days after contact with chickenpox won't make you any more likely to become infected. If you do get chickenpox, the anti-viral drug aciclovir may help prevent serious infection in you and your baby.

TWINS, OR MORE

Women aged 35–40 are the most likely to have twins. Sometimes this is because they have produced two eggs, both of which have been fertilised. Fertility treatment with drugs to stimulate the ovaries increases the chance of multiple pregnancy and older women are more likely to have had such treatment.

But enough of medical problems. Now to preparing for your baby's arrival.

CHAPTER THIRTEEN

Preparing for the birth and your baby

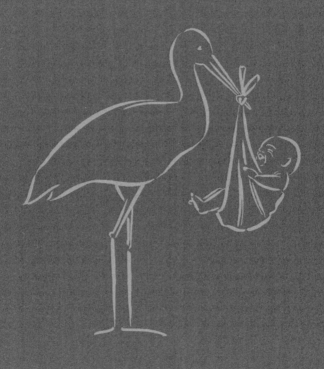

Preparing for a baby can be a delightful experience, especially if you've been waiting some time to get pregnant. As well as choosing equipment and, perhaps, making a room ready, you'll need to ensure you have everything to hand that you'll want by you in labour. It's a good idea to think ahead about who will be with you during labour and who will help out afterwards. And if you intend returning to work, you need to make arrangements for child-care.

BABY EQUIPMENT

Choosing equipment is important, as well as a lot of fun. It can also be expensive! You may have more spending power than a younger woman if you've advanced in your career, or have worked for some years and have saved, or if your partner earns well. However, there's no need to spend a lot. What is important is to have safe equipment, which makes buying second-hand or accepting hand-me-downs not always such a good idea. All major equipment should have a current safety standard mark.

Cot. On no account must you use a cot painted with lead-containing paint (see page 37). So don't use an old family heirloom unless you're assured by the giver – or a test – that the paint is lead-free. Nor must cot bars be too far apart or your baby could get his or her head stuck. And, of course, the cot must be sturdy, the drop-down sides in good working order, and the base sound.

Carrycot/baby seat/car seat. Modern portable baby seats are easier to handle and carry than old-fashioned carrycots and some double as car seats. If you're planning on using a second-hand one, check the handle is well fixed and the harness secure. It's best to play safe by buying a new car seat and having any necessary anchorage points fitted professionally.

Pram/buggy. Safety and strength are most important. Weight may be relevant too if you want to pop it in and out of the car or take it up and down stairs.

WHAT YOU'LL NEED DURING THE BIRTH

Collect together the things you'll need during labour. Some ideas include:

- Nightie (more practical than pyjamas).
- Slippers – ones with non-slippery soles and which don't come off easily.
- Cardigan or other bed-jacket.
- Dressing gown.
- Paper tissues, bath gear – including a face flannel to cool your face if necessary – and other toiletries.
- Magazine, book, or Walkman with headphones.
- Massage oil for labour.
- Hair-band.
- Sanitary towels and pants for afterwards.
- Small change or cards for telephone calls and money for the hospital shop or trolley.
- Addresses and telephone numbers, with writing paper, etc. Remember, though, that you can't take a mobile phone into hospital because it would interfere with some of the vital electronic medical equipment.

ARRANGING FOR COMPANY IN LABOUR AND HELP AT HOME AFTER THE BIRTH

Think who you'd most like to take you to hospital and be with you in labour. For many women this is their partner but some choose their mother or sister, a friend, or even their ante-natal teacher.

Although you can't know yet how much help you'll need in the early days after the birth, it's worth making some plans. Discuss with your partner how much time he can take off, and together with him and your close relatives and friends work out who'll be available to look after you and do the shopping, cleaning, cooking and so on when you get home. You may choose to have paid help – a cleaner, mother's help, au pair or even a maternity nurse – in which case you'll probably need to select that person now.

MAKING OTHER DOMESTIC ARRANGEMENTS

Some women stock the freezer, fridge and cupboards or even freeze ready-cooked meals ready for the week or so after the birth. It's worth enquiring whether any local shops have a telephone ordering and home delivery service; a few large supermarkets now operate on the Internet.

DECIDING ON CHILD-CARE IF YOU INTEND AN EARLY RETURN TO WORK

Now's the time to think about the various sorts of child-care and decide what appears best.

Choices include negotiating care by a family member in their home or yours; taking your child to a childminder – preferably a registered one; booking into a day nursery; or employing a nanny at home. If you work part-time at home, an au pair or mother's help might be best.

RASPBERRY LEAF TEA

Red raspberry leaf tea or tablets taken during the last three weeks of pregnancy is said to 'tone' the womb, make contractions more effective, allow a faster, less painful birth and reduce bleeding. It's considered safe, though I know of no proof that it helps. However, cows about to calf seek out raspberry leaves if they're available!

Make the tea by pouring 600ml (1pt) of boiling water over 25g (1oz) of dried or 50g (2oz) fresh raspberry leaves. Cover and steep for ten minutes, then strain and keep up to two days in the fridge. Have a cup a day from 3–6 months, then three a day up until labour. During labour, drink a cupful each hour unless you've been told to have sips of fluid only.

MASSAGING YOUR VULVA

Some women believe that regular massage around the vaginal opening in the vulva in the last few weeks of pregnancy, together with gentle stretching of the opening, makes the area more supple and helps prevent tearing during labour. Using a little massage oil (see page 81) makes this easier. This can be done alone or with your partner.

PLANNING A SPECIAL BIRTH ENVIRON-MENT

Many women remember every detail of their labour and baby's birth for years, if not for ever. You may decide to make your labour particularly memorable by decorating your birthing room at home – or even, if possible, in hospital. You could, for example, have favourite flowers, photographs, pictures or posters, or special lighting, music or scented candles. You might want to have drinks and snacks available for you (unless medically inadvisable) and your birth companion. Or you might like to have some much-loved poetry read to you.

Some women arrange to labour – or even give birth – in a specially constructed pool of warm water.

And others think ahead about celebrating their baby's birth with a blessing, prayer or song, even if they plan a christening or other dedication later.

The next thing after all the months of planning and preparation is the birth itself.

CHAPTER FOURTEEN

The birth itself

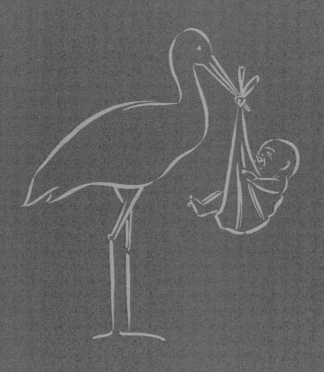

M any women make the process of birth their special focus throughout pregnancy. And the emergence of a baby after months in the womb remains one of life's great miracles.

LABOUR AND BIRTH – WHAT TO EXPECT

Your baby will come when ready, but doctors generally recommend not waiting beyond 42 weeks. If you feel the time's about right and you'd like to get going, try the age-old methods of frequent intercourse (because prostaglandins in semen can encourage labour that is imminent), or frequent orgasm or nipple stimulation (which raise your oxytocin level and have a similar labour-inducing effect).

Every woman's labour is different. Your midwife and doctor will give you some idea beforehand of whether it's likely to go smoothly, but that's all. Don't forget you can change your birth plan (see page 65) at any time, right up to and during labour, if you find you want to do things differently. Events may overturn your plans anyway.

Most women make their way to hospital during the first stage of labour – as their contractions gradually ease open the neck of the womb.

ACTIVE BIRTH

It's best not to go to bed during labour unless you have to – or unless it's the middle of the night and you want to get some rest early in labour. Contractions are most effective when a woman is upright and on the move. Many women also find them less painful if they move around to adopt whatever position feels most comfortable at the time. This may mean leaning forwards and supporting some of your weight with your hands on something in front of you. You can lean forwards like this while standing up, or when kneeling with your knees bent either at right angles or fully flexed.

If you have backache, try getting on all fours and gently rocking your pelvis with small up and down movements of your lower back. Lowering yourself on to your elbows may help even more.

If your baby needs electronic monitoring, it may be possible to have a machine with a long enough lead for you to be out of bed and relatively mobile.

BIRTH POSITIONS

Kneeling up – either on the labour bed or on the (clean and covered) floor – is an excellent position to adopt for contractions later in the first stage, as the second stage approaches. Leave it

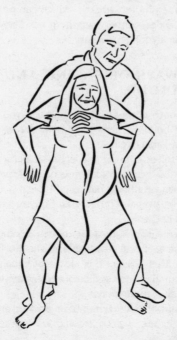

much later and you may find it difficult to get on to your knees! Some women adopt a semi-squatting position with each contraction in the second stage, with a helper behind supporting them under their armpits. A few supple ones find squatting best, though this position can make labour a little too rapid for safety.

The advantage of kneeling or squatting is that your trunk is upright yet you can also easily adjust your position by leaning forwards and shifting your pelvis around. So as the baby comes down your birth canal in the second stage, not only does gravity help the descent, but you can make sensitive movements of your pelvis from side to side, or by bending your body at the hips, whichever makes that particular contraction easier to bear and use effectively.

Remaining upright has been proven to make birth safer for most babies, and women less likely to tear or need an episiotomy. It also tends to shorten labour – which can be an advantage for the average older mother for whom it's likely to be relatively longer than in a younger woman.

OTHER WAYS OF EASING AND DEALING WITH LABOUR

- Ask your birth companion to massage you in whatever way feels most helpful – light stroking at the base of the spine is often remarkably effective.
- Make yourself as comfortable as possible, for example by keeping warm, and using a cold flannel on your forehead, or a hot or cold pack on your lower back.
- Use the breathing and other relaxation exercises you learned in ante-natal classes.
- You can use a TENS (trans-cutaneous electrical nerve stimulation) machine if one's available in the hospital, or if you've hired one. This delivers tiny electrical impulses through pads fixed to your abdomen and back and some women find it helps them manage labour pains.
- Your midwife or doctor may offer pain relief with a mask delivering a mixture of gas (nitrous oxide or laughing gas) and air;

pethidine injections; or an epidural anaesthetic. Some women have a 'mobile' epidural which paralyses only the pain nerves. This allows them to walk around.

SHOULD YOU TRY TO AVOID AN EPISIOTOMY?

It's obviously better not to have an episiotomy (a cut made towards the back of the vaginal opening just before the baby's head is delivered) unless really necessary. However, it's sometimes vital to get a baby who is short of oxygen out faster (perhaps with a forceps or vacuum extractor), or to prevent tearing of the mother's perineum.

Experienced midwives are skilled in facilitating the smooth, controlled delivery of a baby's head so it stretches the vaginal opening evenly and slowly. You can help prevent unnecessary tearing by remaining upright during the second stage. Some people think drinking raspberry leaf tea (see page 113) and massaging the vulva (see page 114) in the last few months of pregnancy and in labour can help to avoid tearing.

COPING IF THINGS DON'T TURN OUT AS EXPECTED

Of course, not every baby is born easily, normally or healthy. Some have a low birth-weight or are unwell and need special care; others take time to settle into life outside the womb and are extra fussy or hard to get to know. Some women need a Caesarean operation. And, tragically, a few babies die.

This is the time to take full advantage of the skilled medical and nursing help you or your baby need. It's important too to accept support from your partner, family and friends and to give yourself time to adjust to things being as they are, not as you expected they would be. You may be interested in a booklet, *What Next?*, from the Birth Defects Foundation (see page 134).

CELEBRATING THE BIRTH

You may feel so exhausted immediately afterwards – especially if labour has been harder or longer than you expected or you needed medical intervention – that all you want is a cup of tea and a sleep. Or you may, like many women, feel wide awake, elated and keen to talk about what's just happened.

Wait until the time is right to celebrate the birth. And if you find yourself feeling low, dejected or even depressed after a few days (see page 126), postpone the celebration until you feel better. There's no hurry – you are the priority.

One of your first steps as a mother is to start feeding your baby. It is also important at this time to remember to look after yourself.

CHAPTER FIFTEEN

Feeding your baby and looking after yourself

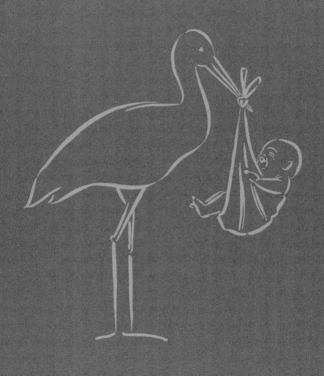

B reast is best for babies and it's wise to aim for four to six months of exclusive breastfeeding and then to continue as long as you and your baby want.

Women in their 30s and 40s are more likely to breast-feed. They tend to be more highly educated and aware of its benefits and also to have more confidence in their own maternal instinct and common sense.

BREASTFEEDING

Breastfeeding provides your child with a real head-start. It also has far-reaching repercussions on a baby's future health – and on yours too. Unlike cows' milk formula, breast milk is the perfect food and breastfeeding has many proven benefits.

BENEFITS TO BABIES:
- Less illness and hospitalisation.
- Fewer infections.
- Fewer allergies.
- Less risk of coeliac disease (digestive problems from cereal gluten sensitivity).
- Less risk of pyloric stenosis (vomiting because of a tight stomach outlet).
- Less risk of meconium ileus (blockage of a new-born's bowel).
- Less risk of appendicitis.
- Less risk of ulcerative colitis and Crohn's disease (inflammatory bowel diseases).
- Less risk of acrodermatitis enteropathica (a scaly skin disease).
- Fewer unexplained cot deaths.
- Less risk of dental decay.
- Better jaw and mouth development.
- Optimal brain development.
- Less risk of diabetes.

- Less risk of cancer.
- Researchers suspect that those breastfed as babies may also be less likely to develop juvenile rheumatoid arthritis, schizophrenia, multiple sclerosis and heart disease.
- Breastfeeding is arguably a more intimate and pleasurable experience than bottle-feeding.

BENEFITS TO MOTHERS:
- Cheaper.
- Useful contraception if you also use the sympto-thermal method. This involves learning how to assess the state of your vaginal mucus and certain other body signs for changes due to impending ovulation. While breastfeeding, this method is most reliable if you learn it from a teacher or follow the instructions in a book on the subject. An electronic ovulation predictor can enhance this method.
- Researchers suspect that women who breastfeed are less likely to develop ovary, womb and pre-menopausal breast cancer, and post-menopausal osteoporosis.
- Breastfeeding is arguably more convenient, satisfying, enjoyable, fulfilling and empowering and provides a more intimate relationship with the baby.

OVERCOMING ANY DOWNSIDES
You may feel embarrassed about showing your breasts in front of certain people, or in public, but you can learn the knack of feeding discreetly.

Breastfeeding needn't be tying and if you want to go out without the baby you can leave expressed milk for someone else to give. It's worth noting that some countries make breastfeeding easier than others. Norway, for example, provides a year's maternity leave at 80 per cent of pay! With this plus other support, 90 per cent of Norwegian women

Breastfed babies tend to sleep less than bottle-feds and to take shorter naps

breastfeed for nine months or more. In contrast, in the UK only 25 per cent of women breastfeed for even four months!

Problems such as sore nipples or uncomfortable breasts are easily overcome if you know what to do.

Breastfed babies tend to sleep less than bottle-feds and to take shorter naps. The biggest downside for many women is having to stop breastfeeding before they or their babies are ready. The commonest reason women give is 'insufficient milk'. Being unable to satisfy a baby is disappointing and frustrating and causes a real crisis of confidence. But studies show that *over 95 per cent of women can provide plenty of milk for their babies*.

So what's their secret?

THE SECRETS OF SUCCESS

Accept that successful breastfeeding is a learned skill. Surprising numbers of women, for example, start off believing their babies need four-hourly feeds. This simply isn't true. Babies don't live by the tick of the clock and may need far more frequent – or longer – feeds than you expect. They also have growth spurts

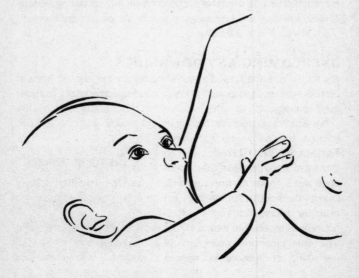

when they are extra hungry and times when they need reassurance from 'comfort sucking' rather than 'food'.

Seek information and support. This is available from skilled professional advisers, from La Leche League leaders and National Childbirth Trust breastfeeding counsellors (see pages 134–135); and, possibly, from other breastfeeding mothers. You can read how to breastfeed successfully in *Breast is Best* (see page 136).

Book into a hospital with a good breastfeeding record. Find out by asking other women, your doctor and hospital staff. Hospitals that encourage breastfeeding can apply for a 'Baby Friendly' award. The top 'Global Award' means the hospital follows all the 'Ten Steps to Successful Breastfeeding' outlined by UNICEF and the World Health Organisation. See how your hospital measures up by writing to the UK Baby Friendly Initiative (see page 135) for their Mothers' Charter leaflet.

BOTTLE-FEEDING

The bottle-feeding woman is lucky in that her helpers are much more likely to be skilled with bottle-feeding than breastfeeding. And no one makes a bit of fuss if she does it in public!

LOOKING AFTER YOURSELF

It's really important to look after yourself now, just as you did before trying to conceive and when you were pregnant. You'll be busy feeding and caring for your baby in the months to come and you'll enjoy it much more if you are fit and well.

FOOD AND DRINK

You need an extra 400–600 calories a day when breastfeeding so choose a highly nutritious diet which supplies plenty of nutrients to replace those in your milk. Now is definitely not the time to go on a low-calorie diet.

Drink as much fluid as your thirst dictates; many breastfeeding women feel thirsty actually during feeds and keep a drink to hand.

It's best to drink alcohol only in moderation; babies take less milk if it tastes of alcohol, and may be fussy afterwards.

EXERCISE
When your doctor gives you the all clear, start doing some daily post-natal exercises (as recommended by the hospital or NCT teacher). But go at your own pace, in tune with how you feel, not according to what other women with similar-aged babies are doing. And don't overdo it, just build your stamina and strength slowly.

Exercise helps tone tummy muscles and makes you feel bright and well. As the weeks pass you can gradually take up some brisker exercise: walking while wheeling your baby along is fine at first; later you could go swimming or join an exercise class, leaving the baby safely nearby, or in a crèche, or with a baby-sitter.

DAYLIGHT AND FRESH AIR
Get outside each day to benefit your bones (see page 30). This is especially important if you are dark-skinned or live in northerly latitudes where the sun's rays are weaker.

BE A NON-SMOKER
If you stopped smoking before or during pregnancy, don't restart now but continue using alternative stress-relieving strategies. This way you'll stay healthier. And if neither you nor your partner smokes, your child is less likely to become ill. Looked at dispassionately, this means less stress for you.

YOUR FIGURE
Breastfeeding doesn't make breasts droopy, as long as you look after them! It's pregnancy that can permanently alter breasts, not breastfeeding. However, it is important to wear a good bra – perhaps also at night – while your breasts are heavier than usual.

FEELING LOW
Whether it's their hormonal changes, tiredness, or the shock of labour and life with a new-born baby, around half of all women feel low when their babies are a few days old. One mother in ten

goes on to suffer from full-blown post-natal depression.

If you feel low, check you're doing basic things like eating a healthy diet, taking exercise (even in the earliest days it's better not to sit or lie down all the time unless you must), and getting some daylight and fresh air every day.

It's also important to have all the practical and emotional support you need, including someone close – such as your partner, mother or friend – who can listen to you over and over again, if necessary, and pick up on your feelings. Don't delay seeking expert help if you continue to feel low or become really depressed. Information and support are also available from the Association for Post-Natal Illness (see page 134).

SEX AND RELATIONSHIPS

The average time after birth for returning to intercourse is around six weeks, though things may continue to feel uncomfortable or strange for some weeks or months until everything is back to normal.

More important than sex is making time to take a loving interest in one another, and to listen, cuddle and be there for each other. It's easier to be a good enough parent to your child if someone gives you some 'tlc' (tender, loving care) yourself. And what better than cherishing and nurturing the relationship that made you parents in the first place?

All this talk about looking after yourself and your baby is fine if you can have a baby or, indeed, want one. But what otherwise?

CHAPTER SIXTEEN

Alternative ways of mothering

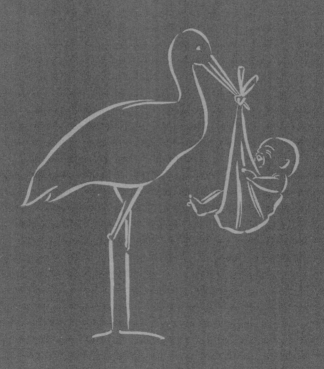

*S*upposing you change your mind and decide not to try for a first baby in your 30s or 40s, or later?

Or what if you find yourself unable to give birth – even with assisted conception and, perhaps, another woman's eggs?

Either way, you still have the opportunity either to become a mother or to use your mothering skills in other ways.

This chapter looks briefly at some possible alternatives.

ADOPTION

You and your partner may consider adopting a child who needs parents. First though, you'll have to be vetted by the adoption agency you choose. And second, you may find you'll need to change your ideas about the sort of child you adopt. Young, healthy babies, for example, are rarely available for adoption, though you may be lucky enough to be offered the chance – and, perhaps, challenge – of adopting an older child, one from another racial group, or one with a physical handicap or learning or behavioural difficulties.

FOSTERING

There's always a need for good foster parents. Fostering may be temporary but sometimes, if the child's natural parents can't or won't take over again, it lasts a long time. Whatever happens, many fostered children and their foster parents forge deep and permanent relationships.

HAVING A STEP-BABY

We can never know what will happen in life or what paths we'll choose to take. If you were to separate from your partner, you might one day meet someone who already has children, in which case you'd become a step-mother. This relationship tends to be easier if the child is very young, or if the mother died, rather than if the parents split up. However, with continued goodwill, love and effort (including skilled empathic listening, plenty of encouragement, and the acknowledgement that you are 'only' a step-mother), even an initially difficult step-relationship can turn out well.

HAVING A SURROGATE MOTHER FOR YOUR BABY (SEE PAGE 134)

Unusual and controversial though it is, surrogacy is officially happening in many western countries today and some believe it may become more acceptable.

Either the surrogate mother becomes pregnant after artificial insemination with a syringe-full of semen from the male half of the couple who want a baby, or eggs are removed from the woman who wants the baby, fertilised in a test tube, and placed in the surrogate's womb.

After the birth, the surrogate hands the baby over to the couple.

This is something of a lottery, though, because some surrogate mothers become so attached to the baby that they refuse to let go. However, surrogacy can sometimes work very well.

BEING A SURROGATE MOTHER FOR SOMEONE ELSE'S BABY

You may even consider becoming a surrogate mother yourself.

DONATING EGGS

There's always a shortage of donated eggs for women who could carry a baby but have no eggs of their own, perhaps because of a premature menopause or because their ovaries have been removed to treat cancer. Obviously it isn't as straightforward to donate eggs as it is sperm. You may also feel you'd like some say in who acts as parents to a child who would genetically be half yours. And you might not like the idea of some fertilised eggs being wasted.

HAVING YOUR BABY ADOPTED

If you are unable, or unwilling, to care for a child but don't want your unborn baby aborted – or your new-born baby fostered until you might one day be able to provide a home – then perhaps your parents or another family might take over, or you could offer your baby for official adoption. You will always be that child's genetic mother and may one day be asked by the adult child to rekindle the relationship that began in your womb and which has remained in your heart ever since.

BEING A GODMOTHER, NEIGHBOUR, GRANNY, AUNT, NURSE, TEACHER, OR ANYONE ELSE WHO SPENDS TIME WITH CHILDREN

Many family roles, jobs, professions and vocations that involve being with children provide the opportunity for some aspect of mothering, whether in the form of practical caring, teaching, sharing time or ideas, encouraging, admonishing, reflecting feelings, or loving.

In a world overflowing with children and with such pressure on so many parents, this sort of 'mothering' is extremely valuable.

WAITING FOR SCIENCE FICTION TO COME TRUE?

Scientists are already working on techniques that may one day permit men to carry a growing fetus inside the abdomen, with the placenta attached to the bowel or other internal organ. And they are developing a technique that could allow a woman to provide the half of the genetic material in a newly conceived baby that has always, until now, been provided by the father. Various other reproductive technologies, including artificial wombs, are also in the pipeline. Strange but true!

MOTHERING OTHERS

To end on a philosophical note, everyone, be they a man or a woman, has repeated chances throughout life to use their learned skills to mother (and father!) others. And you'll mother others best if you can mother yourself properly ... and allow yourself to accept the love that others can give.

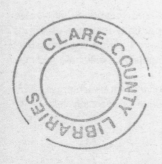

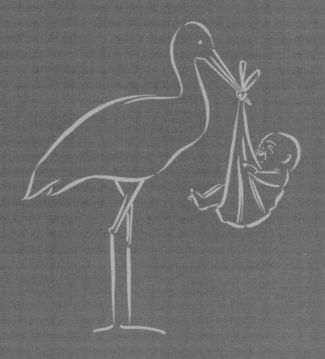

USEFUL ADDRESSES

Action for Pre-Eclampsia (APEC) 31–33 College Road, Harrow, Middlesex HA1 1EJ (Tel: 01923 266778).

Active Birth Centre www.activebirthcentre.com; 25 Bickerton Road, London N19 5JT (Tel: 020 7281 6760).

Action on Pre-eclampsia www.apec.org.uk; 84–88 College Road, Harrow, Middlesex HA1 4HZ (Tel: 020 8427 4217) – provides information and support for pre-eclampsia.

Association for Post-Natal Illness www.apni.org; 145 Dawes Road, Fulham, London SW6 7EB (Tel: 020 7386 0868).

Birth Defects Foundation www.birthdefects.co.uk; BDF Centre, Hemlock Business Park, Hemlock Way, Cannock, Staffordshire WS 11 7GF (Tel: 01543 468888).

BLISS www.bliss.org.uk; 68 South Lambeth Road, London SW8 1RL (Tel: 0870 770 0337) – provides information and support for parents who have, or have had, a baby in special care.

British Agencies for Adoption and Fostering www.baaf.org.uk Skyline House, 200 Union Street, London SE1 0LX (Tel: 020 7593 2000).

Caesarean Support Group – see National Childbirth Trust.

CHILD www.child.org.uk; Charter House, 43 St Leonard's Road, Bexhill-on-sea, East Sussex TN40 1JA (Tel: 01424 732361) – self-help support network for those with fertility problems.

Childlessness Overcome Through Surrogacy (COTS) www.surrogacy.org.uk; COTS, Lairg, Sutherland IV27 4EF (Tel: 0844 414 0181).

Down's Syndrome Association www.downs.syndrome.org.uk; (Tel: 020 8682 4001).

Ectopic Pregnancy Support Group c/o the Miscarriage Association (see below).

Foresight Charity for Preconceptual Care 28 The Paddock, Godalming, Surrey GU7 1XD (Tel: 01483 427839).

International Association of Infant-Massage www.iaim.org.uk; Sparsholt Road, Barking, Essex IG11 7YQ (Tel: 07816 289 788) – trains infant massage instructors who teach parents.

ISSUE, The National Fertility Association www.issue.org.uk;

(Tel: 09050 280 300).

La Leche League BM 3424, London WC1N 3XX (Tel: 0845 120 2918) – provides breastfeeding support and information. If you're on the Internet, visit the LLL International website at: www.lalecheleague.org

Life www.lifeuk.org.contact.html; Tel: 01926 421587. – gives practical help and counselling to women with an unplanned pregnancy, post-abortion counselling; and accommodation for homeless pregnant women.

Meet-a-Mum Association (MAMA) www.mama.org.uk; 376 Bideford Green, Linslade, Leighton Buzzard, Beds LU7 2TY (Tel: 01525 217064) – offers contacts for all mothers and support for post-natal depression.

Miscarriage Association c/o Clayton Hospital, Northgate, Wakefield WF1 3JS (Helpline: 01924 200799, Mon–Fri, 9–4).

National Childbirth Trust www.nctpregnancyandbabycare.com; Alexandra House, Oldham Terrace, London W3 6NH (Tel: 0870 444 8708); breastfeeding line 0870 444.

National Childbirth Trust (Maternity Sales) Ltd catalogue from 239 Shawbridge Street, Glasgow G43 1QN (Tel: 0141 636 0600).

National Egg and Embryo Donation Society (NEEDS) (Tel: 0161 276 6000) – provides potential donors with information.

Paintmakers Association James House, Bridge Street, Leatherhead, Surrey KT22 7EP (Tel: 01372 360660) – leaflet, *How to remove old lead paint*.

Quit (Quitline 0800 00 22 00) – for stop-smoking help.

Stillbirth and Neonatal Death Society (SANDS) 28 Portland Place, London W1N 4DE (Tel: 020 7436 7940).

Twins and Multiple Birth Association (TAMBA) www.tamba.org.uk; (Tel: 0800 138 0509).

UK Baby Friendly Initiative 20 Guilford Street, London WC1N 1DZ – makes awards to hospitals with a good record of facilitating breastfeeding.

BOOKS

Getting Pregnant, by Robert Winston (Pan)

The Mothercare New Guide to Pregnancy and Babycare, by Dr Penny Stanway (Conran Octopus)

Easy Exercises for Pregnancy, by Janet Balaskas (Frances Lincoln)

Breast is Best, by Drs Penny and Andrew Stanway (Pan)

Coping With Your Premature Baby, by Dr Penny Stanway (Orion)

OTHER PRODUCTS

Aromatherapy massage oil for pregnancy: from the Active Birth Centre, 25 Bickerton Road, London N19 5JT (Tel: 020 7281 6760).

Essential oils of high quality: from Wessex Impex Ltd, Stonebridge Farmhouse, Breadsell Lane, St Leonard's, East Sussex TN38 8EB (Tel: 01424 830659).

Electronic ovulation monitor: 'Persona', from large branches of Boots.

'Sea-Bands': elastic wrist bands to counteract nausea; from chemists and travel shops or Sea-Band UK, Church Walk, Hinckley, Leicestershire LE10 1DW (Tel: 01455 251020).

Supplements: suitable for women while waiting to conceive and during pregnancy; available from pharmacies and other retail outlets.

Multi-vitamin and multi-mineral supplements – examples include 'Pregnacare' (Vitabiotics), 'Pregnancy' (Boots), 'Pregnancy Pack' (Health Plus) and 'Foresight' (Cantassium).

Essential fatty acid supplement – 'Efanatal' (Efamol Ltd).